Y0-EGI-212

PREVENTION'S BEST™
America's #1 Choice for Healthy Living

PAIN-FREE LIVING FOR SENIORS

355 Ways to Turn Off Pain without Radical Procedures

By the Editors of *Prevention* Health Books

RODALE

ST. MARTIN'S
PAPERBACKS

Material in this book appeared previously in *Seniors Guide to Pain-Free Living*
(Rodale Inc. 2000), *Age Protectors* (Rodale Inc. 1998), *Nature's Medicines*
(Rodale Inc. 1999), and Prevention's *Healing with Motion* (Rodale Inc. 1999).

Prevention's Best is a trademark and *Prevention* Health Books is a registered
trademark of Rodale Inc.

PAIN-FREE LIVING FOR SENIORS

Cover Designer: Anne Twomey
Book Designer: Keith Biery

ISBN 0–312–97877–4 paperback

Printed in the United States of America

Rodale/St. Martin's Paperbacks edition published May 2001

St. Martin's Paperbacks are published by St. Martin's Press, 175 Fifth
Avenue, New York, NY 10010.

10 9 8 7 6 5 4 3 2 1

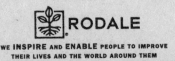

RODALE

WE INSPIRE AND ENABLE PEOPLE TO IMPROVE
THEIR LIVES AND THE WORLD AROUND THEM

Notice

This book is intended as a reference volume only, not as a medical manual. The information given here is designed to help you make informed decisions about your health. It is not intended as a substitute for any treatment that may have been prescribed by your doctor. If you suspect that you have a medical problem, we urge you to seek competent medical help.

Contents

PART ONE

Feeling Your Pain

In ancient times, pain was an outright mystery. Doctors attributed it variously to possession by demons, excess fluids in the body, the wrath of the gods, or simply failing to live a devout life. And their treatments were tied to their diagnoses: exorcism, bloodletting, purging, sacrifices.

Frightening stuff for sure—and not very effective either.

Today we have a much better handle on the real causes of pain. Plus, we're much better prepared to control, or at least reduce, most forms. In fact, these days there's no shortage of successful treatments, from conventional therapies, like using potent pain medications or applying heat and cold, to some strategies that might surprise you, like exercising more, changing your diet, and just improving your attitude.

In the chapters ahead, we'll help you understand pain and show you how to treat it so it doesn't put the whammy on your life. Armed with that knowledge, you can begin to put your pain demons to rest—succeeding in ways of which your ancient ancestors could only dream.

An Introduction
to Pain and Aging

In his heyday, Edward H. Gibson was a star attraction for just one reason. He never—except for an occasional headache—felt an ache or pain in his life. Not that he didn't try. In a fit of rage, he once broke his nose by banging it on a piano. In another instance, he was accidentally struck in the head with a hatchet. Nothing hurt him.

In the 1920s, Gibson made much of this distinction, touring on the vaudeville circuit as "The Human Pincushion." Twice a day, dressed only in shorts, he would come out on stage and ask a volunteer from the audience to stick as many as 60 pins into him in a single performance. Then, in front of the audience, Gibson would calmly pull the pins out one by one.

Never feeling pain, like Edward Gibson, might seem like a dream. But it isn't. Without the ability to sense pain, you'd be more prone to burns, infections, and injuries—and worse.

"Generally, the few people who are born without the ability to perceive pain don't live very long," says Stephen

W. Harkins, Ph.D., professor of gerontology, psychiatry, psychology, and biomedical engineering at the Virginia Commonwealth University in Richmond. "Pain plays an important part in self-protection and self-preservation. Without it, a person tends to take great risks that others wouldn't."

Too Much of a Good Thing?

So a certain amount of pain is vital for survival. But instead of being a useful sensor that keeps you out of harm's way, pain can become the equivalent of an annoying car alarm that howls incessantly for no apparent reason. Over time, unrelenting pain in the back, hips, and other parts of your body takes its toll, causing depression, sleep disturbances, mobility problems, and other difficulties that can diminish the quality of your life, says Randall Prust, M.D., medical director of both the Center for Pain Management at El Dorado Hospital and the Pain Medicine Center at Tucson General Hospital, both in Tucson, Arizona, and author of *Conquering Pain.*

In fact, persistent, unrelieved pain is the most common complaint among older Americans, according to the American Geriatrics Society. But before you indict Father Time or think only the elderly suffer, you should know this: Aging probably has little to do with your pain.

"Many people—patients, families, and even some health-care providers—believe that pain is just an expected consequence of aging, and if it is happening to you, you have to learn to live with it because nothing can be done to stop it. That's not true at all," says Keela Herr, R.N., Ph.D., a pain researcher and associate professor of nursing at the University of Iowa College of Nursing in Iowa City. "Chronic pain is not an inescapable part of growing older."

Lifestyle, not the aging process, is the real underlying culprit that triggers many of the painful diseases— such as arthritis, osteoporosis, and sciatica—that become more common as people get older, doctors say.

"We tend to pretend that we don't have to do anything to maintain our health, and that eventually catches up with us," says Margaret A. Caudill, M.D., Ph.D., codirector of the department of pain medicine at the Dartmouth-Hitchcock Medical Center in Manchester, New Hampshire, and author of *Managing Pain Before It Manages You.*

Potent Pain Preventers

Inactivity, poor nutrition, smoking, drinking too much alcohol, and being overweight are just a few of the things that can aggravate any ache in your body, Dr. Prust says. But, as doctors point out, all those are lifestyle factors that you can change, too.

"It is not too late to prevent existing aches and pains from getting worse, nor is it too late to prevent the onset of new aches and pains," says Risa Lavizzo-Mourey, M.D., director of the Institute on Aging and chief of the division of geriatric medicine at the University of Pennsylvania Medical Center in Philadelphia.

Here are a few potent, natural lifestyle changes you can incorporate right now that will help you prevent or even relieve aches and pains throughout your body.

"These are lifestyle changes that will help in the long run," Dr. Prust says. "The pain won't go away tomorrow, but if you stick with these lifestyle changes, you'll gradually start feeling better and better, and stronger and stronger."

Keep moving. Regular physical activity is one of the best things you can do to relieve or prevent incessant pain,

Dr. Prust says. In fact, the less you do, the more intensely you'll feel pain.

"When you're sedentary, your muscles turn into butter. And when that happens, your bones lose all of their structural support. That's going to make your pain feel worse," he says. "It's like a building: The bones are the columns, and the muscles are the brick and mortar. Without the brick and mortar, the building will collapse."

In addition, regular activity bolsters bloodflow to areas that do hurt, helping the body heal itself faster, Dr. Prust says. Try to do an activity you enjoy—no matter if it's golf, tennis, swimming, walking, or gardening—for at least 20 minutes 3 or 4 days a week.

"You have to pick something you like; that's the key," he says. "Personally, I love water exercises. The water is very soothing, and I think people like it because it takes the weight off their joints. I tell people to just start walking in the pool every day. That is the simplest exercise you can do." Check with your local pool to find out if it offers water stretching, yoga, or aerobics classes.

Eat the right foods. Without good nutrition, you'll be more prone to chronic aches and pains, Dr. Prust says.

"You need every cell in your body to be in tip-top shape in order to fend off pain," he says. "If you don't eat a well-balanced diet, your body won't have all of the building blocks it needs to do that."

He suggests eating a daily diet that includes 6 to 11 servings of breads, cereals, rice, and pastas; 3 to 5 servings of corn, carrots, and other vegetables; 2 to 4 servings of oranges, bananas, strawberries, and other fruits; 2 to 3 servings of milk, yogurt, and other low-fat dairy products; and 2 to 3 servings of meat, poultry, fish, eggs, nuts, or dry beans. Remember, don't go overboard. A portion doesn't have to be huge—one banana or one slice of bread counts as a serving.

Call in reinforcements. Glucosamine, a sugar that is one of the body's natural building blocks, and chondroitin, another natural chemical, are an important dynamic duo that can keep your joints pain-free, Dr. Prust says. These two chemicals, which naturally diminish in the body as you age, help maintain cartilage and other vital connective tissues surrounding your joints.

Specifically, glucosamine helps repair damaged cartilage tissue, and chondroitin moisturizes cartilage so that it doesn't become brittle, he says. To picture how these chemicals work, imagine that your cartilage is a well-manicured lawn. As you age, you may be more prone to get crabgrass or dry, brown spots on that lawn. Glucosamine helps your body get rid of the crabgrass, and chondroitin eliminates dry, brown spots. As a result, your cartilage stays healthy, and your joints remain pain-free.

You'd have to eat far too much food to get enough glucosamine and chondroitin in your diet, so supplements are your best bet. Look for 500-milligram tablets of glucosamine sulfate and 400-milligram tablets of chondroitin sulfate. The dosage depends on your weight. If you weigh up to 110 pounds, Dr. Prust recommends taking two tablets of glucosamine and two tablets of chondroitin daily; 110 pounds to 200 pounds, take three tablets of each daily; over 200 pounds, take four tablets of each a day. These supplements can be taken with or without food, but it's a good idea to take the entire dosage at a single meal simply because it helps you remember to do it. It will be 2 to 6 months before you notice a difference, he says.

Stop smoking. Smoking is one of the worst things that you can do if you are in chronic pain, Dr. Prust says. Nicotine, the active ingredient in tobacco, causes blood vessels to clamp down, cutting off the flow of oxygen and nutrients to the nervous system. Nicotine also may block the release of endorphins, the body's natural painkilling hormones. People who smoke use more narcotics to relieve pain than nonsmokers do.

"I have patients who smoke who can literally feel the pain intensify every time they take a puff," he says. "If there was ever a reason to quit, there it is."

Although smoking is a difficult addiction to break, there are plenty of ways to do it successfully. For starters, Dr. Prust suggests you try nicotine patches and gums—two of the most effective methods—which are available over-the-counter.

Decaffeinate your life. Like smoking, drinking too much caffeine slashes bloodflow to your joints and can heighten your sense of pain throughout your body. Limit yourself to no more than two cups of regular coffee or three cups of regular tea a day, Dr. Prust says. You can drink as many decaffeinated beverages as you like since most of the caffeine has been removed. Certain foods, like chocolate and sodas, also contain caffeine, so read food labels carefully.

Limit alcohol use. Some people believe they can drink their pain away, Dr. Prust says. But in reality, alcohol damages nerves, diminishes the effectiveness of pain medication, and disrupts the body's repair mechanisms.

"Even in small quantities, alcohol can cause problems if you have chronic pain," he says. "Any nerves that are damaged by alcohol are probably going to be raw, inflamed, and hurt like heck. There is no question that having more than two drinks a day is going to harm nerves and increase your susceptibility to chronic pain syndromes."

Shed extra pounds. Excessive weight puts unnecessary strain on most joints in the body and can trigger pain, Dr. Prust says."If you have to use a lot of energy just to maintain all the fat in your body, then you're not going to have a lot of energy to fight pain," he says. "If you're overweight, that's like carrying around a 30-, 40-, or 50-pound bag of dog food with you everywhere you go. That makes it much likelier that you're going have a lot of aches and pains."

Small changes in your eating habits and activities can make a big difference in your weight, Dr. Prust says. So to kick-start your weight-loss effort, begin your meals with a fibrous food like an apricot, a slice of whole-grain bread, or a raw carrot. Fruits, vegetables, beans, and grains are packed with nutrients and usually have few calories. Fiber also adds bulk to your diet, so your stomach fills up faster and you eat less. As for activity, look for ways to burn extra calories, like parking farther away from your destination.

Reach out to others. If you have too much time on your hands, you'll probably dwell on your aches and feel worse. So stay as socially active as you can. Volunteer at your library or another agency in need. Take a class at a community college. Join a band.

"Social activity helps take your mind off the pain," Dr. Prust says. "The most common time for patients to have pain is first thing in the morning or at night when other people aren't around. So companionship or social activity of some kind is necessary to divert the brain from the pain."

Imagine that there's no pain. Imagery is a powerful mind/body technique that can help keep aches and pain from creeping up on you, says Dennis Gersten, M.D., a psychiatrist and medical director of the Gersten Institute for Higher Medicine in Cardiff-by-the-Sea, California, and author of *Are You Getting Enlightened or Losing Your Mind?*

To try it, take a couple of deep breaths, then imagine that you are holding a ball of mercury (the silver liquid found in thermometers) in your hands and that it can draw pain out of your body like a magnet. Now imagine that any pain developing in your body—even if you don't feel it right now—is sucked into this magnetic ball of mercury and disappears into the ball. Then let the ball, which is now full of pain, dribble onto the floor and flow out of sight.

Do this for 1 minute twice a day to keep pain under wraps, Dr. Gersten suggests.

The Two Sides of Pain

Believe it or not, pain has its good side. Bang your knee, smash your finger in a doorjamb, or cut yourself on the hand, and that instantaneous pain sends you a clear message: Ouch! Stop! Tend to this injury now!

It's called acute pain. To soothe it, you might apply ice to the swelling, use an antibiotic ointment, or cover the wound with an adhesive bandage. In a few minutes or a few days, the wound heals and the pain disappears.

Even when the problem is more serious, such as a kidney stone, pain is doing a good deed. This acute, excruciating pain is telling you to do something about it—in this case, seek immediate medical care. Once the crisis passes, the pain withers away.

But acute pain has a demonic twin. Chronic pain lingers on long after the body has healed. In some cases the pain persists for years or even decades. Often doctors can find no underlying cause for it. Chronic pain affects more than 50 million people in the United States. Nearly one in five Americans takes pain medication to combat it.

And the reasons for its prevalence and tenacity are compelling and mysterious.

Acute Pain Jangles Your Alarm Bells

For most of us, all pain seems the same. Whether it stings, burns, throbs, or grates, we know only two things: It hurts, and we want it to go away. But before you can begin to soothe any discomfort, it's important to know more about the differences between acute pain and chronic pain, and how they are treated.

"Acute and chronic pain are quite distinct," says Robert N. Jamison, Ph.D., director of the pain-management program at Brigham and Women's Hospital in Boston and author of *Learning to Master Your Chronic Pain*. Acute pain is a message that something is wrong and you need to tend to it. Chronic pain really isn't very helpful. It's a signal that's hard to turn off.

Acute pain is normally predictable. It has a beginning, a middle, and an end. Rest, a bit of heat or cold on the injury, an over-the-counter analgesic like ibuprofen, and the passage of time are usually enough to get you through the worst of it.

"People usually recover from acute pain in a reasonably limited time span," says Margaret A. Caudill, M.D., Ph.D., codirector of the department of pain medicine at the Dartmouth-Hitchcock Medical Center in Manchester, New Hampshire, and author of *Managing Pain Before It Manages You*.

Whether it's sharp pain from a needle prick or dull pain from an upset stomach, pain signals are relayed to your spinal cord. From there it passes through a complex series of specialized nerve cells that act like gates. If the pain isn't particularly bothersome, these gate cells can diminish or even cancel the signal before it gets to the brain. But if

When to Go to a Pain Clinic

When all else fails, a comprehensive pain-treatment center often can do wonders to eliminate or dampen persistent pain, says Harris McIlwain, M.D., a pain-management expert in Tampa, Florida, and coauthor of *Winning with Chronic Pain*.

You'll be cared for by a team of physicians and other health professionals who together can develop a pain-management program that's right for you. A typical team might include doctors who specialize in treating the brain, muscles, bones, and joints. You might also be treated by an occupational therapist, a physical therapist, or even a dentist. This multidisciplinary approach allows doctors to fully evaluate the causes of your pain and offers you the best chance of finding relief, Dr. McIlwain says. Treatments range from simple stretching exercises to highly complex surgery.

When is it time to go? When you're not getting the pain relief you need from your family doctor, chiropractor, or other health-care provider. But because Medicare may pay for only some of the costs of treatment at a pain clinic, *before* you agree to any care, be sure to double-check which services will be covered.

the pain is intense enough, the signal passes from the spinal cord to the brain, says Randall Prust, M.D., medical director of both the Center for Pain Management at El Dorado Hospital and the Pain Medicine Center at Tucson General Hospital, both in Tucson, Arizona, and author of *Conquering Pain*.

A portion of the brain called the thalamus sends out two messages. One travels to your cerebral cortex, the thinking part of the brain, which assesses the damage that is causing the pain and spurs the body's repair mechanisms into action. The second message is sent back to the injury or wound, ordering the pain receptors to stop sending out messages. To ensure that this order is carried out, the body also releases morphinelike hormones called endorphins and enkephalins that help dampen pain. Of course, if the injury is severe—like a broken leg—the pain receptors will likely disregard this order and continue sending out intense distress signals that will encourage you to seek medical care.

Acute pain is complex, but in most instances it does its job and then fades away. When it doesn't, the real troublemaker, chronic pain, can set in.

Chronic Pain: The Ache That Runs Amok

"Chronic pain is garbage in the brain. It is not useful information that the body can use in any meaningful way," says Norman J. Marcus, M.D., medical director of the Norman Marcus Pain Institute in New York City and the Princess Margaret Hospital Pain Treatment Center in Windsor, England, and author of *Freedom from Chronic Pain*.

Unlike acute pain, which lasts only a few seconds to a few weeks, chronic pain can last for months, years, or even decades. Although it may begin as acute, useful pain—a symptom warning you to rest an inflamed back muscle, for instance—over time chronic pain transforms itself into a disease, much as literature's gentle Dr. Jekyll turned into venomous Mr. Hyde.

Chronic pain plunders your vitality, shatters your self-esteem, and consumes your life. Yet, strangely enough, a medical examination may reveal that the body has healed and that the physiological changes, such as increased heart rate, that accompany acute pain have returned to normal, Dr. Marcus says. But that doesn't mean the pain is a figment of your imagination. It is quite real.

"If you feel pain, you've got pain," says Nelson Hendler, M.D., director of the Mensana Clinic in Stevenson, Maryland, one of the nation's first pain clinics. "The reason you have chronic pain is you still have something wrong with you."

But what that "something" could be remains elusive. Doctors simply aren't sure how or why the body's nervous system runs amok and causes chronic pain.

"According to conventional wisdom, when pain lasts more than 3 months, it shifts from the acute phase into the chronic phase. What happens during that transition? We don't know," says Jeffrey Ngeow, M.D., associate attending anesthesiologist and former director of the pain-management program at the Hospital for Special Surgery in New York City.

Nerve damage or diseases such as arthritis and diabetes can contribute to the development of chronic pain. But it also can occur without a known injury or disease. What's clear is that the gateways regulating pain sensation are blocked open, allowing nerves to continue sending their torturous messages on a fast track to the brain. Plus, all of the emotional and psychological responses to acute pain are magnified when it becomes chronic, leading to a cycle of insomnia, fatigue, irritability, anger, and sadness that can aggravate your condition.

Doctors also know that many of the standard treatments for acute pain—rest, heat, cold, and medication—aren't always the best choices for relieving chronic pain.

While rest is beneficial for acute pain, it actually can make chronic pain worse, Dr. Marcus says. Excessive rest can lead to flabby muscles, frail bones, substantial weight gain—and *more* chronic pain. So stay as active as you can.

In the long run, painkillers are often ineffective against chronic pain, Dr. Marcus says. Instead of relieving your torment, these drugs can actually lower your pain threshold. "Pain medication is useful for chronic pain only if you're using it to improve and facilitate activities of daily living," he says. "If you're taking a medication that doesn't help you function any better, what good is it?"

So what *does* combat chronic pain? Plenty, including exercise, relaxation techniques, and other therapies and remedies we'll discuss in this book. It's never too late to do something about it.

Where Does It Hurt?

Even under the best of circumstances, communication is a fragile thing. And under the stress and strain of medical care, communication often crumples as easily as a dry leaf. Yet when you're in pain, nothing—absolutely nothing—is more critical than finding the right words to help your doctor understand your agony.

"Communicating with your health-care provider about your pain is the most important thing you can do to take an active role in your own care. It's vital for you to make your doctor or nurse aware of exactly what is going on," says Keela Herr, R.N., Ph.D., a pain researcher and associate professor of nursing at the University of Iowa College of Nursing in Iowa City.

Bridge the Communication Gap

Your doctor can't feel your pain. Neither, for that matter, can your friends or relatives. It isn't like a rash, which everyone can see and touch. Nor does pain feel the same to all people. A sprained ankle may hardly bother one person but can be unbearable to another. And although grimaces, twinges, and other nonverbal expressions of pain can give doctors a pretty good idea of how much you hurt, they really won't know unless you speak up. In fact, if you are stoic enough, your pain can be virtually invisible to others.

"Far too many Americans needlessly endure pain because they don't talk to their doctors about it. They either mistakenly believe that their doctors can't do anything about it, or they simply don't know how to describe their pain," Dr. Herr says. "Many times they feel that nurses and doctors, because of their experience, know when someone hurts. And if something could be done, they would be doing it without being asked. Unfortunately, that's not true. In many instances, nothing will be done unless you bring your pain to their attention."

But many people are reluctant to do that. In fact, more than one in four people surveyed said there have been times when they wanted to talk to a doctor about a health problem but were reluctant to do so. Yet in that same survey, 9 out of 10 doctors agreed that serious medical problems such as pain could be averted if patients were willing to talk more freely. And two out of every three doctors said that it is difficult to treat patients who are hesitant or too embarrassed to talk about their health problems.

"Doctors aren't mind readers. We have to be told when you are in pain, what your pain is like, and what affects it. And the only person who can accurately do that is you," says Paul Blake, M.D., a pain-management expert and outpatient services director at Meridian Point Rehabilitation Hospital in Scottsdale, Arizona. Here are some ways you can bridge the communication gap and help your doctor understand your pain.

Before You Go

Chart a course. Take a few minutes *before* you visit the doctor to sketch out an agenda of what you would like to discuss during the appointment, suggests Judson J. Somerville, M.D., an interventional pain-management specialist in Laredo, Texas. It could simply be a written list of your five major symptoms and concerns. At the appointment, hand your list to the doctor as he walks into the examination room.

"Frequently, what happens is that the doctor will speak very fast, throw a lot of questions at you, and then move on to the next patient. A list of symptoms is something that might slow the doctor down a little bit so that he will spend some extra time with you," he says.

The list will help you organize your thoughts so that you won't forget to mention a bothersome symptom or side effect of your treatment. From the doctor's standpoint, a written list—typewritten, if possible—will help him quickly address your concerns and spot telltale symptoms that might refine your diagnosis and treatment.

Make your first shot count. A typical person gets only about 18 seconds to explain a medical problem before the doctor interrupts with questions.

To make the most of that time, you need to state what you expect out of the visit clearly and concisely, says Margaret A. Caudill, M.D., Ph.D., codirector of the department of pain medicine at the Dartmouth-Hitchcock Medical Center in Manchester, New Hampshire, and author of *Managing Pain Before It Manages You*.

So before your appointment, take some time to imagine that your doctor has just walked into the examination room. What would you like to say in two or three sentences? Write that down. Now imagine how you'd like your doctor to reply to you. Do you want advice, reassurance, compassion, information, or a combination of these things? Now try rewriting your opening statement so that it includes a clear request for what you expect your doctor to do for you. You might, for example, say, "I'm scared, so I would appreciate it if you would reassure me" or "I don't expect miracles, but I would like some advice about coping better with flare-ups without using drugs."

"Many times people come in and say, 'My pain is worse. It's terrible. I can't take it anymore.' End of story. They don't come right out and ask for what they really want," Dr. Caudill says. "It is very helpful to know right up front exactly what a patient is looking for."

Take five. Anticipate the five questions your doctor is most likely to ask you about your pain, suggests Michelle Bricker, M.D., director of the University Center for Pain Medicine and Rehabilitation at Hermann at the University of Texas Medical Center in Houston. If you can, jot down your responses to the following questions and take them with you when you visit your doctor.

- Where do you feel the pain, and what does it feel like?
- When did you first notice the pain you are experiencing now?
- Is there anything—such as changing your body position—that seems to make the pain feel better or worse? If so, what?
- Does the pain come and go, or is it persistent?
- Does it hurt more in the morning than in the evening or vice-versa?

If you're prepared for these questions beforehand, it can save time and help you clearly communicate your needs, Dr. Bricker says.

Keep track of your aches. Often it is difficult to convey to your doctor in a short office visit how much the pain really hurts in your everyday life. So keep a pain diary, and

Spotting Emergency Pain

If you whack your head on a kitchen cabinet, it hurts. Most pains are like that. They're easily explainable and quickly go away without treatment. But certain pains should never be ignored, says Stuart Farber, M.D., a geriatrician, pain-management expert, and clinical assistant professor of family medicine at the University of Washington in Seattle. Seek immediate medical attention if:

- You have pain in the chest that spreads into your neck, jaw, or left arm. This symptom also may be accompanied by shortness of breath, dizziness, nausea, vomiting, sweating, or generalized weakness.
- You develop a sudden, severe headache accompanied by numbness, dizziness, tingling, or you have difficulty walking, seeing, speaking, or swallowing.
- You develop sudden back or lower abdominal pain and feel light-headed or dizzy.
- You have constant abdominal pain that is in the lower right area of your belly or that lasts for more than an hour and is accompanied by fever.
- You have painful urination accompanied by back pain, blood in your urine, or the urge to urinate more frequently.
- You have any other new, unexplainable pain that lasts more than a week.

take it in with you each time you see your physician, Dr. Caudill suggests. Record your pain level on a 0-to-10 scale (10 being the worst pain you can imagine) three times a day at regular intervals, such as morning, noon, and bedtime. Do this for at least 3 months, Dr. Caudill says, and you might start noticing patterns of pain that you can point out to your doctor.

Keep time on your side. If you suspect that you'll need more than a 15-minute appointment to discuss your aches and pains, let the doctor's receptionist know it when you make your appointment, Dr. Caudill suggests. That way, you and your doctor will feel less hurried.

In the Exam Room

Be succinct. Whenever you are describing your pain, stick to the pertinent facts, suggests Stuart Farber, M.D., a geriatrician, pain-management expert, and clinical assistant professor of family medicine at the University of Washington in Seattle. Avoid straying off the subject. If you're describing how you injured your elbow while playing tennis, for instance, avoid going into the details about the match or or asking the doctor for tennis tips. Instead, focus on how the injury occurred and how you feel now. So you might say, "Every time I play tennis, I end up with a sharp pain in my elbow for days afterward. It starts the day after a game and will last for a week or so. It even hurts, for example, whenever I lift my coffee cup." That approach will grab your doctor's attention, Dr. Farber says.

Let your doc feel it, too. Just saying "It hurts" isn't going to help your doctor understand your pain. Be specific—let the doctor know precisely how the pain is disrupting your life, Dr. Farber suggests. So if you have a sore ankle and it is preventing you from doing daily activities such as walking, playing tennis, puttering in the garden, or even doing household chores, speak up.

"When you break down pain into a personal experience so that the physician can understand how it is really affecting you, it's a much more persuasive motivator for the doctor to help you do something about it," Dr. Farber says.

Know the lingo. The more accurately you can describe your pain, the better the chances are that your doctor can help find relief, Dr. Farber says. Use simple words like *stinging, burning, throbbing, aching, cramping,* or *jabbing* that can help the doctor pinpoint the problem.

A sharp, stabbing pain in your legs and back that goes all the way down to your toes, for example, will probably need to be treated differently than a burning, scalding pain that begins in your hip and travels down the front of your thigh. "Details like that can help your doctor understand the mechanism of your pain and what can be done about it," Dr. Farber says.

Pick a target. If you have more than one ache or pain, zero in on the most bothersome one first, suggests Norman J. Marcus, M.D., medical director of the Norman Marcus Pain Institute in New York City and the Princess Margaret Hospital Pain Treatment Center in Windsor, England, and author of *Freedom from Chronic Pain*.

"If you tell the doctor that you hurt everywhere, you can forget about getting good care. Everything doesn't hurt everywhere in exactly the same way," he says. "You're better off saying something like 'Yes, I do have a lot of aches and pains, but this one is unique, and here's why it's unique. This pain feels like somebody is jabbing in my lower back. It comes on when I do this or when I don't do that. It doesn't respond to medication the way my other pains do.' Information like that will give your doctor something to work with."

Make sure you understand the doctor. If an explanation or procedure puzzles you during the exam, ask your doctor for clarification. Otherwise, he will assume that you understand what is going on, Dr. Blake says.

You might say something like "I still don't quite get what you're trying to tell me. Can you explain it again?"

"Some people are reluctant to ask their physicians to repeat instructions they don't fully understand," Dr. Blake says. "But you have to keep in mind that your physician is there to educate you as well as treat you. So it's okay to keep asking questions until you fully grasp it."

Make sure the doctor understands you. Similarly, if your doctor doesn't seem to understand you, ask him to repeat what you just told him about your aches and pains, Dr. Somerville says. If it doesn't match what you said, try restating your problem until the doctor gets it.

"Just take one step back and say, 'Somehow, doctor, I'm not conveying to you what is wrong with me. Is there some way I can explain it to you better or differently?'" he says. "That way the doctor won't feel as if you're attacking him and then react defensively to your comments."

Say, "Show me." Ask your doctor to use pictures, drawings, and other visual aids that will make your pain and its treatment easier to comprehend, Dr. Somerville suggests.

Get it in writing. Ask your doctor for pamphlets, step-by-step instructions, or other written materials. These handouts can help you understand your condition and help you recall exercises and other techniques he suggests for relieving your aches and pains, Dr. Blake says.

Before You Leave

Let it all simmer. After your appointment ends, take a few minutes to sit down in the waiting room to jot down notes or go over any written materials you were given during the visit. If you don't understand something, particularly the diagnosis, testing procedures, treatment, or even when you are supposed to return for a follow-up visit, ask a nurse for clarification, Dr. Somerville suggests. If you're still confused after that conversation, ask to speak briefly with the doctor.

Know when to connect. Physicians, like most of us, tend to be busier at certain times of the day than others. So be sure to ask a nurse when would be the best time to telephone your doctor if you have a question or need advice between appointments, Dr. Somerville suggests. If you phone and leave a message, let the doctor know when you'll be at that number so he can contact you. If you have access to a computer, you also might ask whether the doctor has e-mail.

Ask for a second opinion. If, after talking to the doctor, you're still uncomfortable about some aspect of your diagnosis or treatment, ask for a second opinion, Dr. Blake says. "There is nothing wrong with getting a second opinion for a complicated problem like pain. You're not necessarily going to hear the same thing from a second doctor. Most doctors won't get upset with you if you ask for another opinion."

If you do ask for a second opinion, be sure to sign a release form before you leave the office and request that your doctor forward a copy of your medical records to the consulting physician.

Adopting
a Pain-Free Attitude

You may not have a choice of when or where you hurt, but you certainly can choose how you react to your pain. And that reaction—that attitude—has as much to do with your pain as any mangled nerve or spasmodic muscle in your body.

"Attitude can make all the difference in the world. If you have a hopeful, self-assured attitude, it helps you feel less overwhelmed or managed by the pain," says Margaret A. Caudill, M.D., Ph.D., codirector of the department of pain medicine at the Dartmouth-Hitchcock Medical Center in Hanover, New Hampshire, and author of *Managing Pain Before It Manages You*. "Attitude really sets the tone of how you perceive the ability to manage the symptoms."

Virtually every negative emotion—fear, depression, anxiety—sparks an incredible biological assault on your nervous system, says Dharma Singh Khalsa, M.D., a pain-management expert in Tucson, Arizona, and author of *The Pain Cure*. Your heart beats faster, your body secretes stress hormones, your muscles tense, your blood vessels constrict, and neurotransmitters in your brain are overly stimulated. As a result, your pain threshold plunges, and your body's ability to counteract your discomfort is diminished.

This suffering often is a self-perpetuating cycle that is hard to break. But you can do it.

Ending Pain Positively

Positive thinking won't make all of your pain go away, but you have more control than you think when you're in the midst of a pain problem. Among other things, a positive attitude triggers the release of endorphins, powerful morphinelike substances in the brain that relieve pain, says Stanley Chapman, Ph.D., a psychologist at the Emory Clinic Center for Pain Management in Atlanta.

In addition, a brighter attitude helps move the pain and suffering from the forefront of your thinking into the background, says Emmett Miller, M.D., who practices in Los Altos and Nevada City, California, and is the author of *Deep Healing: The Essence of Mind/Body Medicine*. And when that happens, a pain that once seemed unbearable might become a mere nuisance.

"Miracles happen when your outlook changes," says Robert N. Jamison, Ph.D., director of the pain-management program at Brigham and Women's Hospital in Boston and author of *Learning to Master Your Chronic Pain*. "If your perception of the pain changes, then the pain itself may actually go down."

Here are a few ways you can foster a pain-free attitude.

Ax the four-letter words. The words *pain* and *hurt* are associated with fear, helplessness, and isolation. So use neutral terms, such as *discomfort* and *sensation*, which imply that you can help yourself and stay active, Dr. Miller suggests. This subtle change can make a huge difference in your attitude.

Take a look at the big picture. Jot down all the things you deeply desire from life, like taking a cruise or spending more time with friends. You'll probably realize that there is much more to your life than just overcoming the pain, and it may have a profound effect on your attitude toward your discomfort, Dr. Khalsa says.

This goal-setting exercise, called psychic clustering, can help you regain control of your destiny and cast off attitudes that have allowed pain to dominate your life, he says.

Visualize the pain disappearing. Visualization, a powerful mind-control technique, can help you dampen pain and reshape your attitude toward it, Dr. Khalsa says. In a study done at a major pain clinic, 20 percent of people with severe chronic pain attained total relief after just 4 weeks of visualization training.

"Visualization literally reprograms the brain and alters perception of pain," he says.

To try it, sit in a quiet place, close your eyes, breathe deeply, and relax as much as possible, Dr. Miller says. As you relax, imagine there's a movie screen in front of you and you can see any part of your body on it. Picture the area that's been having unpleasant sensations. If you wish, picture the letters P-A-I-N on that screen.

As you look at that shape on that screen, notice what color it is, or give it a color that matches the sensation. See the color clearly. See the size and shape of this area. Is it a bright color or dull? Are its borders smooth or irregular? Does it look flat or bumpy? Is it the same color throughout, or does it vary in color? As you continue to relax, let the color and the image fade. As this happens, the unwanted sensation will continue to fade along with it, becoming less and less as you slip into a deep, comfortable state of peace.

Now imagine that you are entering the deepest part of

your mind, Dr. Miller says. Picture it as a control room with switches and knobs that control the amount of awareness of any sensation. By adjusting these controls, you turn down the sensations in your body so they fade far, far away. Notice that there is a knob that controls your awareness of the sensation that was projected on the screen. Grasp this knob now and begin to turn it down so the sensation disappears, as though dissolving into a cloud of peace and relaxation.

Do this for 10 to 15 minutes twice a day, Dr. Miller suggests.

Turn to meditation. Meditation is one of the best ways to rise above pain and forge a positive attitude, Dr. Khalsa says. It increases your "mental energy," so your brain can launch an effective counterattack against the pain. In addition, meditation allows you to slip into a state of absolute calm, called the sacred space, that triggers regeneration and healing of the mind, body, and spirit.

Find a quiet, comfortable spot where you won't be disturbed. Close your eyes and take several deep, relaxing breaths. If any thoughts intrude, let them drift away, and redirect your attention to your breathing.

To help focus the physical energy of your brain, press the tip of your left thumb on your forehead, between your eyebrows, he suggests. This is the area of the brain where your highest thought processes occur. Then, with your thumb still pressing on your forehead, make a fist, but leave your little finger extended. Grasp your extended little finger in the palm of your right hand, and extend the little finger of your right hand. Hold this position for 3 minutes as you continue to breathe deeply. Now lower your hands; you should feel more focused and aware of your body.

Keep breathing deeply through your nose—about 8 to 10 breaths per minute. As you do, focus your attention on an area in your body that hurts. Notice how the discomfort waxes and wanes, Dr. Khalsa says. Now focus on areas of your body that do not hurt. Pay attention to the comfort you feel there, and realize that this sensation is just as real as the pain. Don't become attached to the comfort or repulsed by the pain. Just accept these sensations as they are. Allow peace of mind and spirit to grow with each breath. And as it does, feel tension, worry, and discomfort wash away.

Do this meditation for 10 to 15 minutes twice a day, Dr. Khalsa suggests.

Accentuate the positive. Affirmations can change how you think about your pain and actually help keep it in check, Dr. Khalsa says. So at least three times a day, take a few minutes to state how you would *like* to feel. You might, for example, tell yourself, "I'm in power. Not my pain."

The more you repeat these affirmations, the more powerful they will become, and the greater the likelihood they'll become a natural way of thinking.

Use your body wisely. Treat pain like money. You have only so much to spend, so you have to decide what is worth spending on, says Eric Willmarth, Ph.D., a pain-management expert and president of Michigan Behavioral Consultants, based in Grand Rapids. Suppose, for instance, you were invited to your niece's wedding. You may be standing a lot and may be in pain afterward. Is that worth it? Probably. On the other hand, if you're invited to a neighborhood block party, you might not want to spend your pain that way. Thinking about activities this way will help you regain a sense of control over your pain, he says.

Flip a switch. Whenever you have a negative thought about your pain, jot it down on a notepad. Take a hard look at that thought. Now think of a rational, positive response to that statement and write that down, Dr. Caudill suggests. You might think, for instance, "I can't do anything because of this pain." Your response might be "If I take frequent breaks, I can still do many things I enjoy." After a couple of weeks, you might find that your negative thoughts have been replaced by positive ones.

"When you're in chronic pain, you tend to think the same negative thoughts over and over again," she says. "Many people who go through this exercise tell me they discover that everything in their lives needn't be black or white."

Carry a trump card. After you've listed your negative thoughts, you'll probably start seeing the same phrases over and over again. If so, jot down five of your most common negative thoughts on one side of an index card. On the other side, write down five replacement thoughts for these negative attitudes. Carry this card with you. When one of these thought pops into your head, pull out the card and use one of the replacement phrases to drown out the negative one, Dr. Jamison suggests.

So if you typically think, "This is unbearable," write that phrase on the card. On the flip side, jot down phrases like "I've gotten through this in the past, and I'm going to get through this again."

Follow the crowd. Socialize. Go to the bowling alley or a nearby coffee shop. On a daily basis get out to where people are, Dr. Jamison says.

"If you have nothing going on except the four walls around you and an ever-present silence, your pain is apt to overwhelm you," he says. "But if you get out and do things that occupy your mind, it will help diminish your discomfort and help you feel more connected with the world." If it's not possible to get out and about, pick up the phone and talk to a friend or get together for a game of cards or lunch. Take up a hobby to help keep your mind active and involved. The Internet can also be a great way to bring the world to you by letting you look up subjects that interest you. You can even chat online with friends and family.

Spot a smile maker. Find a heartwarming experience in each day, Dr. Willmarth suggests. Watch a toddler picking a dandelion. Take time to contemplate a rainbow.

"The more ammunition you can give yourself for developing a positive attitude, the better off you'll be," he says. "Train yourself to observe beauty, humor, compassion, and other good things around you."

Exercise your funny bone. Laughter is a potent weapon against pain, Dr. Jamison says. It relaxes tense muscles, decreases the production of stress-related hormones, and distracts your mind from the pain. So if you're having a particularly rough day, imagine how your favorite comedian would describe it. This will help you laugh it off. Reserve a portion of your refrigerator or bulletin board for cartoons and funny pictures or sayings. Stockpile a library of humorous writings and videos you can turn to when your pain flares up.

"Humor helps a lot. Pain is so deadly serious and makes you so miserable that it is hard to distance yourself from it," he says. "But laughter can renew your sense of why life is worth living."

The Good and Bad of Drugs

War is hell. You should know; you're waging a battle against pain. And just like soldiers on a real battlefield, you need the best weapons in your arsenal to win. In this war, that sometimes means painkilling drugs. But like any weapon, a drug can be self-destructive as well as useful. Even the ancient Greeks recognized that drugs were a double-edged sword. Their word for drugs, *pharmakos*, meant both "remedy" and "poison."

But you have an important ally on your side: knowledge. Doctors and pharmacists now know far more than ever about the limitations and dangers of drugs. And by the time you finish this chapter, so will you. This knowledge will help you overcome fears and misconceptions you may have about using these medications as part of an overall battle plan to conquer your pain.

To Prescribe or Not to Prescribe

Drugstores boast a dizzying array of pain medications—some available over-the-counter, others by prescription.

Which is better? Which is cheaper? Which is safer?

Here's the rule of thumb: When you have a minor pain such as a simple headache, bruises, or aches from straining, treat it first with acetaminophen as directed on the label, says Mark Baugh, Pharm.D., a pharmacist at San Diego Hospice and author of *Sports Nutrition: The Awful Truth.* Then, if that isn't working after 24 hours, stop taking it and try a nonsteroidal anti-inflammatory drug (NSAID), the most common of which is ibuprofen. The over-the-counter strength is 200 milligrams. If you take the recommended amount—two tablets—you're getting 400 milligrams, which is equivalent to the lowest dosage available by prescription. If that isn't working within 24 hours, then the next logical step is to see a doctor for a prescription.

Know Your Weapons

Today's arsenal of prescription pain relievers includes everything from aspirin to Cox-2 inhibitors, a new generation of NSAIDs. Also, medications developed for other uses, such as anticonvulsants, antidepressants, and corticosteroids, can relieve some types of pain. The following drug profiles show common options, along with their hidden benefits and side effects or risks.

Acetaminophen

WHAT IT IS: Available over-the-counter, acetaminophen alleviates pain by inhibiting the production of prostaglandins, hormonelike substances that lead to swelling and help transmit pain to the brain. It's best for minor aches and pains, pain with bruising, and muscle pain.

ACTIVE INGREDIENT (COMMON BRAND): Acetaminophen (Tylenol).

COMMON SIDE EFFECTS: None.

SAFE USE: Don't exceed package directions—too much can cause liver and kidney damage. If you suspect that you've taken too much, contact the nearest poison information center. Do not drink alcohol if you'll be taking more than two doses of acetaminophen.

HIDDEN BENEFITS: Research suggests that when a single dose is taken on a daily basis, acetaminophen may reduce the risk of ovarian cancer by half.

NOT RECOMMENDED FOR: Heavy drinkers or people with liver damage. If you consume alcoholic beverages, consult your physician before using acetaminophen since it is hard on the liver.

SPECIAL HINTS: Keep your acetaminophen out of damp places, including your bathroom medicine cabinet. Heat and moisture cause it to break down.

Many heavily advertised names can be more expensive; check into store brands. Don't waste your money using this medicine for the swelling of arthritis—it isn't as effective against inflammation as other medications. Save it for headaches and other minor aches and pains.

Anticonvulsants

WHAT THEY ARE: Anticonvulsants are medications prescribed to control seizures. They can be helpful for nerve pain, especially burning, stabbing pains due to diabetic neuropathy and postherpetic neuralgia.

ACTIVE INGREDIENTS (COMMON BRANDS): Carbamazepine (Tegretol) and gabapentin (Neurontin).

COMMON SIDE EFFECTS: Clumsiness, dizziness; light-headedness; drowsiness; nausea; vomiting; irregular, pounding, or unusually slow heartbeat; and chest pain.

Take Pains to Ask These Questions

Here are the three most important questions to ask your doctor about a medication, according to Isaiah Florence, M.D., director of the Center for Pain Management at Englewood Hospital and Medical Center in Englewood, New Jersey.

- Does this interact with my other medications?
- What are the side effects?
- What can I expect this medicine to accomplish for me?

SAFE USE: Take this medicine as prescribed for a specified pain only. Do not use it to treat minor discomforts. These agents are not simple analgesics and should not be taken casually.

HIDDEN BENEFITS: Carbamazepine has been used to treat the acute phase of schizophrenia when other medicinal agents have failed.

NOT RECOMMENDED FOR: People who are allergic to tricyclic antidepressants and those with liver or bone marrow disease should avoid taking carbamazepine.

SPECIAL HINTS: Keep this medicine out of damp places, including your bathroom medicine cabinet. Heat and moisture cause it to break down.

Combination Drugs

WHAT THEY ARE: These nonprescription pain relievers have more than one ingredient. Caffeine is added to enhance the absorption of the aspirin or acetaminophen, so it gets to your brain—and stops pain—faster. The aspirin-based brands work best for arthritis, while those containing acetaminophen are best for tension headaches.

ACTIVE INGREDIENTS (COMMON BRANDS): Acetaminophen, aspirin, and caffeine (Excedrin Extra-Strength); aspirin and caffeine (Anacin); and acetaminophen and caffeine (Aspirin-Free Excedrin).

COMMON SIDE EFFECTS: Abdominal cramps or stomach pain, heartburn or indigestion, nausea and vomiting, slowed blood-clotting time (for medicines containing aspirin), jitters and trouble sleeping (for medicines containing caffeine).

SAFE USE: Since these drugs contain caffeine, they may taint the results of certain blood tests. Before having medical testing, tell your doctor that you're taking these medications.

HIDDEN BENEFITS: Research suggests that a single daily dose of acetaminophen may slash the risk of ovarian cancer in half.

Aspirin is approved by the FDA to reduce the risk of subsequent strokes and adverse cardiovascular events. It reduces the risk of death from heart attacks, prevents second heart attacks, and diminishes the risk of heart attack in people with angina. Preliminary evidence suggests aspirin users have fewer lung and breast cancers. One animal study found that aspirin may reduce the risk of getting a form of hereditary colon cancer.

NOT RECOMMENDED FOR: Drugs containing acetaminophen are not recommended for heavy drinkers or people with liver damage. If you consume alcoholic beverages, consult your physician before using this drug, especially because both acetaminophen and alcohol are hard on the liver. Medications containing aspirin are not recommended for people with asthma, nasal polyps, high blood pressure, bleeding disorders, severe liver or kidney disease, stomach ulcers, or history of hemorrhagic stroke.

SPECIAL HINTS: To prevent gastrointestinal side effects, take with meals.

Corticosteroids

WHAT THEY ARE: Corticosteroids are prescription medications that provide relief of inflammation. They provide pain relief by reducing swelling, itching, redness, and allergic reactions. They work best for arthritis, cancer pain, and surgical pain, especially when there is inflammation.

ACTIVE INGREDIENTS (COMMON BRANDS): Betamethasone (Celestone), cortisone (Cortone Acetate), dexamethasone (Decadron), prednisolone (Predalone 50), and prednisone (Orasone).

COMMON SIDE EFFECTS: Increased appetite, indigestion, restlessness, nervousness, trouble sleeping.

SAFE USE: Because steroids may lower your immune function, infections may be harder to treat. Make sure to talk to your doctor if you develop symptoms of an infection, such as fever, difficulty breathing, or pain in your kidneys or bladder. To prevent stomach problems, take steroids with food. Don't drink alcohol while taking steroids.

HIDDEN BENEFITS: None.

NOT RECOMMENDED FOR: People with active tuberculosis, fungal infections, herpes infection of the eyes, or peptic ulcer disease.

SPECIAL HINTS: Since side effects occur with prolonged use, avoid using these medications for long periods of time. Sometimes steroids can be taken every other day or at varying doses to lessen side effects. Check with your doctor to see if this is right for you. Avoid people with influenza, chickenpox, or measles and those who have recently taken an oral polio vaccine. During the time that your immunity is compromised by steroids, you could be susceptible to these illnesses, even if you already had them once.

Cox-2 Inhibitors

WHAT THEY ARE: Hailed as the new generation of non-steroidal anti-inflammatory drugs, Cox-2 inhibitors promise to relieve the pain of arthritis without causing the gastrointestinal problems of older NSAIDs. Cox—short for cyclooxygenase—is an enzyme that controls the production of hormonelike substances called prostaglandins that

The Keys to the Medicine Chest

If you're confused when choosing pain pills, here's a quick primer to popular options.

- Buffered. An antacid has been added to the medicine to protect your stomach. Experts say buffering doesn't do much to save your stomach, but it does help the pill dissolve faster.
- Enteric-coated. These pills are less likely to cause stomach upset because they dissolve in your intestines instead of in your stomach. But they also take about 15 minutes longer to start working.
- Time-release, delayed-release, or extended-release. These medications are scientifically designed so some of the medicine dissolves fast, then the inner core is released over an extended period of time. They don't provide the quick pain-relief punch of other analgesics.

lead to swelling and transmit pain to the brain. There are two types of this enzyme: Cox-1 and Cox-2. Cox-1 controls prostaglandins that help to create the protective mucus of the stomach, so if it's suppressed, damage to the stomach can result. Cox-2 regulates prostaglandins that cause inflammation and pain, so if it's suppressed, you'll have less pain. While older NSAIDs block both Cox-1 and Cox-2, Cox-2 inhibitors block only the prostaglandins you want to block, the ones that cause pain.

ACTIVE INGREDIENTS (COMMON BRANDS): Celecoxib (Celebrex) and rofecoxib (Vioxx).

COMMON SIDE EFFECTS: Gastrointestinal bleeding, skin rash, weight gain, fluid retention.

SAFE USE: If you are prone to stomach ulcers, don't use Cox-2 inhibitors until the ulcers are completely healed and your doctor says it's okay.

HIDDEN BENEFITS: They're gentler on the gastrointestinal system than other pain medications, and they may slow the progression of cancer and Alzheimer's disease. Unlike other NSAIDs, Cox-2 inhibitors don't appear to increase the risk of uncontrolled bleeding.

NOT RECOMMENDED FOR: People who have had reactions, such as wheezing hives or allergies, after taking aspirin or other NSAIDs. Also not recommended for those who are allergic to sulfonamides.

SPECIAL HINTS: These drugs are expensive. Use them only if you have drug-induced ulcers and can't take NSAIDs.

Narcotics/Opioids

WHAT THEY ARE: Potent drugs that suppress activity in the central nervous system and relieve pain. These drugs are available by prescription only. They are usually reserved for moderate and severe pain, especially bone and muscle pain, cancer pain, and pain during surgery or times when other medications haven't worked for unrelenting pain.

ACTIVE INGREDIENTS (COMMON BRANDS): Codeine, hydrocodone, fentanyl (Sublimaze), oxycodone (Procolan), morphine (Duramorph), methadone (Dolophine), propoxyphene (Darvon), hydromorphone (Dilaudid), and meperidine (Demerol).

COMMON SIDE EFFECTS: Dizziness, light-headedness, drowsiness, nausea, vomiting, constipation.

SAFE USE: Don't combine narcotics with alcohol or other medicines, such as antihistamines, that slow down the nervous system.

HIDDEN BENEFITS: These medications can also reduce anxiety.

NOT RECOMMENDED FOR: People with severe asthma or those with fluid in their lungs from congestive heart failure.

SPECIAL HINTS: Dry mouth is a common side effect. To combat it, try chewing candy or gum, melt ice in your mouth, or use a saliva substitute.

Nonsteroidal Anti-Inflammatory Drugs (NSAIDs)

WHAT THEY ARE: These drugs—available by prescription and over-the-counter—relieve inflammation by halting the production and release of prostaglandins, hormonelike substances that lead to swelling and help transmit pain to the brain. They work best for mild to moderate pain accompanied by swelling. They are commonly used to treat both types of arthritis, stiffness, joint pain, bursitis, tendinitis, sprains, and strains.

ACTIVE INGREDIENTS (COMMON BRANDS)—PRESCRIPTION: Indomethacin (Indocin), nabumetone (Relafen), sulindac (Clinoril), flurbiprofen (Ansaid), diflunisal (Dolobid), piroxicam (Feldene), etodolac (Lodine), meclofenamate (Meclomen), fenoprofen (Nalfon), naproxen (Naprosyn), ketoprofen (Orudis), tolmetin (Tolectin), and diclofenac (Voltaren).

ACTIVE INGREDIENTS (COMMON BRANDS)—NONPRESCRIPTION: Ibuprofen (Advil, Motrin-IB, Nuprin), ketoprofen (Orudis KT), and naproxen (Aleve).

COMMON SIDE EFFECTS: Abdominal or stomach cramps, diarrhea, drowsiness, dizziness, light-headedness, headache, heartburn, indigestion, nausea, vomiting, high blood pressure. Since gastrointestinal damage from NSAIDs can occur at any point, short-term use isn't necessarily safer. In fact, long-term use may actually allow gastric mucous membranes to adapt, reducing the chance of stomach problems.

SAFE USE: Don't exceed dosage recommended in package directions—taking too much increases chance of side effects. Never mix NSAIDs with the cancer medication methotrexate (Mexate), which is sometimes prescribed to treat psoriasis and rheumatoid arthritis. This combination can be fatal.

HIDDEN BENEFITS: NSAID use may offer protection against Alzheimer's disease and colorectal cancer.

NOT RECOMMENDED FOR: People with gastrointestinal, liver, or kidney problems or those taking high blood pressure medication. NSAIDs should not be combined with alcohol, because they can increase stomach bleeding, or diuretics, because they can cause an increased risk of kidney failure.

SPECIAL HINTS: Take with a full 8-ounce glass of water. To avoid irritation after swallowing, remain upright for 15 to 30 minutes after taking it. Take with food to alleviate gastrointestinal side effects.

Salicylates

WHAT THEY ARE: These prescription and nonprescription drugs are used to relieve swelling, stiffness, and joint pain. They do this by halting the production and release of prostaglandins, hormonelike substances that lead to swelling and help transmit pain to the brain. They work best to ease symptoms of both types of arthritis, headaches, muscle aches, and dental pain.

ACTIVE INGREDIENTS (COMMON BRANDS)—PRESCRIPTION: Salsalate (Disalcid) and choline/magnesium (Trilisate).

ACTIVE INGREDIENT (COMMON BRANDS)—NONPRESCRIPTION: Aspirin (Bayer, Bufferin).

COMMON SIDE EFFECTS: Abdominal cramps, pain, or discomfort; indigestion; heartburn; nausea; vomiting; high blood pressure.

SAFE USE: Call your doctor if you notice a ringing or buzzing in your ears or headaches. These may be signs that you're taking too much of this medicine. Do not take for more than 10 days in a row without consulting your doctor.

HIDDEN BENEFITS: Aspirin use is approved by the FDA to treat strokes and may prevent future cardiovascular events. It reduces the risk of death from heart attacks, helps prevent second heart attacks, and reduces the risk of heart attack in people with angina. It prevents ischemic strokes, the kind that happen when blood clots clog the

(continued on page 46)

Concerns about Drug and Herb Combinations

In general, herbs cause fewer side effects than drugs. But they're still powerful medicines capable of interacting with other medications. Jennifer Brett, N.D., a naturopathic physician and chairperson of botanical medicine at the University of Bridgeport College of Naturopathic Medicine in Connecticut, offers these three rules for safe herbal healing.

1. Don't use herbs with drugs that have similar ingredients or that act on the body in similar ways. For instance, don't combine willow bark or aspirin with an anticoagulant, such as warfarin (Coumadin).
2. Don't take herbs and other medications or supplements at the same time; they might interact with one another. Your best bet is to separate herbs from other medications by at least 2 hours.
3. Avoid herbs that increase or decrease the amount of time it takes other medications to be absorbed in your body. Licorice, for example, lengthens the time it takes to clear prednisone from the body.

Here are 11 of the most widely used herbs, along with their known drug or supplement interactions.

- Black cohosh. May interfere with effects of low-dose oral contraceptives or hormone replacement therapy.
- Garlic. Can intensify the effect of blood thinners like warfarin (Coumadin).
- Ginger. May inhibit the effectiveness of heart medication, anticoagulants, and diabetic medications.

- Ginkgo. Do not use with antidepressant MAO-inhibitor drugs, such as phenelzine sulfate (Nardil) or tranylcypromine (Parnate), aspirin or other nonsteroidal anti-inflammatory medications, or blood-thinning medications, such as warfarin (Coumadin).
- Ginseng (Panax). Can interact with phenelzine and other MAO inhibitors; don't take with coffee or caffeinated beverages, antipsychotic drugs, or hormone treatments.
- Kava kava. Intensifies the effects of other central nervous system drugs, including alcohol, antidepressants, and antihistamines.
- Licorice. Can interfere with hormone therapy; can lengthen time it takes to clear prednisone from the body; avoid if you take drugs that already leave you prone to potassium loss (thiazide diuretics).
- St. John's wort. Do not use with antidepressants; may increase photosensitivity effect of sulfa drugs or antibiotics like tetracycline.
- Uva-ursi. May irritate bladder when taken with acidic agents, like fruit juice or supplemental vitamin C.
- Valerian. Can intensify the effect of sleep-enhancing or mood-regulating medications such as diazepam (Valium) or amitriptyline (Elavil).
- Willow bark. The active ingredient is related to aspirin and can interact with blood-thinning medications such as warfarin (Coumadin); may interact with barbiturates or sedatives such as aprobarbital (Amytal) or alprazolam (Xanax); can cause stomach irritation when consumed with alcohol.

arteries that supply blood to the brain. Preliminary evidence suggests aspirin users have fewer lung and breast cancers. One animal study hinted that aspirin use may reduce the risk of developing a form of hereditary colon cancer. It may also prevent cataracts.

NOT RECOMMENDED FOR: People with asthma, high blood pressure, bleeding disorders, severe liver or kidney disease, ulcers, or history of hemorrhagic stroke.

SPECIAL HINTS: Smell aspirin (and products containing aspirin) before you take it. A vinegar smell means it's breaking down and should be replaced.

Tramadol

WHAT IT IS: This medication is prescribed to relieve severe pain, particularly after surgery. It works on the brain to decrease pain, and it's best used for moderate to severe pain.

ACTIVE INGREDIENT (COMMON BRAND): Tramadol (Ultram).

COMMON SIDE EFFECTS: Abdominal or stomach pain, anxiety, confusion, nervousness, dizziness, sleep trouble, diarrhea, constipation, nausea, vomiting, excessive gas, dry mouth, skin flushing, headache, heartburn, hot flashes, itching, skin rash, loss of appetite, loss of energy, sleepiness, sweating.

SAFE USE: Take this medication precisely as instructed by your physician.

HIDDEN BENEFITS: Side effects are less likely than with other drugs.

NOT RECOMMENDED FOR: People who are allergic to narcotic medications.

SPECIAL HINTS: Don't take more than 300 milligrams daily.

Tricyclic Antidepressants

WHAT THEY ARE: Prescribed to ease depression, these drugs can also alleviate pain, probably by affecting the part of the brain that controls messages between nerve cells. They're most often used for postherpetic pain, diabetic neuralgia, and other conditions resulting in nerve damage.

ACTIVE INGREDIENTS (COMMON BRANDS): Amitriptyline (Elavil), imipramine (Tofranil), and doxepin (Sinequan).

COMMON SIDE EFFECTS: Dizziness, drowsiness, dry mouth, headache, increased appetite, nausea, tiredness, weakness, unpleasant taste, weight gain, accentuated memory loss.

SAFE USE: These medicines may cause sun sensitivity. Stay out of direct sunlight, or at least wear protective clothing, sunblock, and sunblock lip balm. Take with food, and take only as directed by your doctor.

HIDDEN BENEFITS: Improved sleep.

NOT RECOMMENDED FOR: People who drink excessive amounts of alcohol or those who have glaucoma. If you consume alcoholic beverages, consult your physician before using this drug.

SPECIAL HINTS: To lessen stomach upset, take this medication with food, even for your bedtime dose.

The Pain-Free Lifestyle

Dust accumulates. Dirty dishes mount. Laundry piles up. Spills happen.

Life goes on—no matter how much pain you feel. And it's important—in fact *vital*—that you make every effort to continue living as full a life as possible, even if you are in pain.

"Cooking, cleaning, shopping—everyday activities can help maintain your body and dampen your pain," says Randall Prust, M.D., medical director of both the Center for Pain Management at El Dorado Hospital and the Pain Medicine Center at Tucson General Hospital, both in Tucson, Arizona, and author of *Conquering Pain*. "We've known that for a long time. Years ago, doctors used to keep patients bed-bound after surgery. As a result, they didn't heal as fast, and they developed more complications and experienced more pain. The same thing can happen if you don't stay active in your everyday life."

In fact, the mundane tasks of everyday living can have an extraordinary impact on pain, says Neal Barnard, M.D., president of the Physicians Committee for Responsible

Medicine in Washington, D.C., and author of *Foods That Fight Pain*. Just staying active around the house helps your body produce natural painkillers called endorphins that are as potent as morphine without causing any of that drug's nasty side effects. In addition, everyday tasks strengthen muscles, ligaments, and tendons surrounding your joints and help make your whole body less susceptible to pain.

People in pain who continue to do everyday tasks also increase blood supply to the areas of their bodies that hurt, Dr. Prust says. And more blood means that more oxygen, vitamins, and other vital nutrients will be available to help heal the underlying cause of the pain.

Draining Pain out of the Brain

But the pain-stopping power of everyday life doesn't end there. It also reverberates in the brain, the organ that actually perceives and reacts to pain.

"What seems mundane and what most of us take for granted—keeping a clean house, doing the grocery shopping—becomes an accomplishment and something to strive for when you are in constant pain. It's part of what keeps you going," Dr. Prust says.

People in chronic pain who, with their doctors' approval, find ways to accomplish these routine tasks usually have a better quality of life than those who don't, says Stanley Chapman, Ph.D., a psychologist at Emory Clinic Center for Pain Management in Atlanta. They develop a hardy "I can do it" attitude that motivates them to do more. The bottom line: The more you accomplish despite discomfort, the more tasks you'll be willing to tackle. The more tasks you tackle successfully, the better your self-esteem. A better self-esteem means less depression and a higher quality of life despite the presence of pain.

Breaking Down the Barriers

Certainly, there are limits. Even light dusting can be a challenge when you are in pain, and there are going to be days when you hurt so much that you won't feel up to doing these everyday tasks. That's fine. The important thing is to do as much as you can as often as you can.

"Nothing is perfect," Dr. Barnard says. "But we all can try to do our best. You can do things despite the pain."

But because you are in pain, you may have to make a few changes in your routine—like using lightweight cookware instead of heavy, cast-iron skillets in the kitchen—in order to get these tasks done. And that's okay, too, says Jan I. Maby, D.O., medical director of the Cobble Hill Health Center in Brooklyn, New York.

In fact, even subtle adaptations in the bedroom, bathroom, or kitchen—that most family and friends probably won't notice—can make a huge dent in your pain and greatly enhance the quality of your life, Dr. Prust says.

"One of my patients is in so much pain that she can't lift her arms above her head," he says. But rather than give up the things she wants to do, she changed the way she does them. Now "every day she gets up, she washes her hair, and she puts on her makeup. It's almost second nature for her to do it the way she is doing it now. She has learned to adapt so that she can continue doing *all* of her normal everyday activities."

Your doctor or an occupational therapist can suggest ways to do tasks that will minimize the pain you feel. But here is a room-by-room compendium of ideas to help you get started.

In the Bedroom

Smooth out the wrinkles. Before you get out of bed, use your feet to smooth the sheets at the bottom of the mattress, suggests Shelia Goodwin, P.T., a physical therapist and clinical director of the Workplace, a rehabilitation center in Birmingham, Alabama. For better accessibility, keep your bed away from walls. Nylon tricot sheets are lightweight, stretch without tugging, and can be put on with one hand. Use a wooden pizza paddle or a large spatula to tuck sheets and bedding under the mattress.

If making a bed is too painful, you can forgo sheets and blankets altogether, Goodwin says. Simply curl up in a sleeping bag on top of the mattress. In the morning, just fold the bag over and stuff it into a closet.

Easy on, easy off. Elastic waistbands eliminate the need for belts and can make pants easier to slip on and off, says Denyse Hernaez, O.T., an occupational therapist at the Hospital for Special Surgery in New York City. Instead of slipping a T-shirt over your head, cut open one side, including the sleeve, and attach hook-and-loop fastener so you can slide the shirt sideways and then fasten it shut. When buying clothing, particularly pullover sweaters, get a size or two too large. It will help make dressing easier.

Reach for a stick. If bending is painful, a dressing stick or a reacher can help you pull up pants, put on pullover shirts, or retrieve hard-to-reach clothes, says Debbie Nakayama, a certified occupational therapist assistant at Christ Hospital and Medical Center in Oak Lawn, Illinois. Dressing sticks and reachers are available at most medical supply stores and through rehabilitation/adaptive equipment catalogs.

Beat the buttons. If you have difficulty using buttons, you can hook a large paper clip over a button and then insert the paper clip into the button hole first to help you work the button into place. Or have someone sew hook-and-loop fastener onto your clothing. For appearance, you can permanently attach buttons to the top side of the hole

(continued on page 54)

Stretch Your Limits

Regular exercise is an important component of the pain-free lifestyle, says Paul Blake, M.D., a pain-management expert and outpatient services director at Meridian Point Rehabilitation Hospital in Scottsdale, Arizona. It helps keep muscles and joints strong and limber and bolsters your pain tolerance.

Always stretch before and after doing any strenuous activity, including housework, Dr. Blake says. In addition, walk, bike, or swim 20 to 30 minutes a day four or five times a week. (It doesn't have to be done all at once.)

Don't neglect strength training, either. If you don't have any equipment, simply lifting common household objects like food cans or milk jugs is a terrific way to strengthen your body and increase your mobility, he says. The following exercises target your arms, shoulders, and lower legs. If you have arthritis or other conditions that affect your muscles, bones, or coordination, consult with your doctor.

Arm raise. Sit in a chair, your back straight. Your feet should be flat on the floor, spaced apart so they are even with your shoulders. In each hand, hold a 12-ounce soup can or a 1- to 2-pound hand weight straight down at your sides, your palms facing inward. Lift your arms out sideways until they are parallel to the ground. Your hands should be slightly in front of your body, not straight out to the side. Hold the position for 1 second. Take 3 seconds to lower your arms until they are straight down by your sides again. Pause. Repeat 8 to 15 times. Rest; do another set of 8 to 15 repetitions. This exercise can also be done standing.

Dumbbell row. Stand next to a sturdy chair or weight bench. With your left leg, kneel on one end of the chair while keeping your right foot flat on the floor. Your right knee should be slightly bent, your back slightly arched.

Support yourself with your left arm. Hold a 1- to 2-pound hand weight in your right hand with your arm down at your side, palm facing in toward your body. Take 3 seconds to lift the weight toward your chest by bending your elbow. Lift it until your elbow is a few inches higher than your back. Hold for 1 second. Take 3 seconds to lower your hand to the starting position. Pause, then repeat until you have done the exercise 8 to 15 times. Rest, then do the same on your other side.

Dip exercise. Sit in a sturdy chair with armrests. Lean slightly forward, keeping your back and shoulders straight. Hold on to the arms of the chair. Your hands should be level with the trunk of your body, or slightly farther forward. Place your feet slightly under the chair, keeping your heels off the ground and resting the weight of your feet and legs on your toes and the balls of your feet.

Using your arms, slowly lift yourself as high as you can, keeping your back straight. Many people won't be able to push themselves off the chair when they first try it. Still, the pushing motion will strengthen your arm muscles even if you can't lift yourself off the chair. Don't use your legs or feet for assistance. Slowly lower yourself back down. Repeat 8 to 15 times. Rest; repeat 8 to 15 times.

Plantar flexion. Stand straight behind a chair or table, holding on to the edge for balance. Your feet should be flat on the floor and spaced shoulder-width apart. Rise on your tiptoes as high as you can; hold for 1 second, then take 3 seconds to slowly lower yourself. Do 8 to 15 times; rest a minute, then do another set of 8 to 15 repetitions.

As you become stronger, do this exercise on your right leg only, then on your left leg only, for a total of 8 to 15 repetitions on each leg. Rest a minute, then repeat.

while using the fastener underneath, Hernaez says. Hook-and-loop fastener can be found in most sewing stores.

Sock it to 'em. If you have difficulty putting on your socks, consider buying a sock aid, Nakayama suggests. To use it, slide your sock onto the sock aid form. Then firmly grasp the ends of the cord and allow the toes of the sock to drop to the floor. Slide your foot onto the shell and pull the sock gently on with the cord. Now remove the aid. Sock aids are also available at many medical supply stores and through rehabilitation/adaptive equipment catalogs.

Horn in. A long-handled shoehorn can help maneuver your feet into your shoes, Hernaez says. Soft cushion inserts or gel soles can prevent aching feet and lessen the strain on your legs and back.

When buying shoes, look for a pair that has hook-and-loop closures, a toe area wide enough to prevent rubbing or crunching of your toes, and heels no more than 1 inch high.

Simplify the essentials. For women, consider sports-style, soft-cup bras. They don't have cumbersome hooks, Goodwin suggests. If a girdle is necessary, look for one that has a zipper or other features so that it can be put on with one hand. If your fingers hurt, wear knee-high stockings. Panty hose require more finger strength and dexterity to put on.

For men, clip-on ties eradicate painful struggles with the Windsor knot, she says.

In the Bathroom

Take a seat. Sitting is preferable to standing in the bathroom, Hernaez says, because it is less tiring and usually less painful. So sit in a chair when brushing your teeth, shaving, or putting on makeup. In the tub, use a bath board or a waterproof lawn chair. When you clean

Pace Yourself

As you do your daily chores, make note of how long it takes for your pain to flare up. When it does, stop and do something easy, like phoning a friend or reading the newspaper, suggests Margaret A. Caudill, M.D., Ph.D., codirector of the department of pain medicine at the Dartmouth-Hitchcock Medical Center in Manchester, New Hampshire, and author of *Managing Pain Before It Manages You*.

Jot down how long it takes for your pain to subside to the point where you feel like going back to your previous chore. For example, if you can fold laundry for 10 minutes before your pain stops you, write that down. If you need 15 minutes to recover, note that too.

Once you've established the working and rest periods you need for the majority of your activities, set a timer, and do an activity for only that amount of time. Then reset the timer and do a restful activity until the alarm goes off. Eventually, you'll probably find that the amount of time you can do an activity without pain will increase, and the amount of time you need to rest will decrease, she says.

Researchers suspect that pacing yourself like this helps relieve pain because you're not pushing yourself to the point of exhaustion. Pacing yourself also can prevent pain from spreading to other parts of your body.

the toilet or bathtub, sit on a stool and use a long-handled scrub brush.

Work up a lather. A shower caddy within easy reach will cut down on the need to bend, twist, or stoop in the shower, Nakayama says. Store liquid soap, shampoo, and conditioner in pump dispensers rather than squeeze bottles. If you insist on using bar soap, consider soap on a rope.

Wring yourself out. After bathing, wrap yourself in a terry cloth robe and allow it to soak up the water as you pat yourself dry, Nakayama suggests. This one-step technique is less painful than the awkward contortions of towel drying.

Crank up the commode. The toilet often is the lowest seat in the house. Sitting down and getting up from such a low point can be tricky if you are in pain. A raised toilet seat with armrests, available at most medical supply stores, can make getting on and off the commode a much easier task, Nakayama says.

Get a grip. Apply cylindrical foam tubing—available at most medical supply stores and through rehabilitation/adaptive equipment catalogs—to combs, toothbrushes, and

Brainstorm Pain Stoppers

Jot down the household chores you normally perform in a week. Check off the three that cause the most pain, says Jan I. Maby, D.O., medical director of the Cobble Hill Health Center in Brooklyn, New York. Now concentrate on the most painful of these three tasks. List any ideas—no matter how offbeat—for minimizing the pain when doing this chore.

If doing laundry is a problem, for instance, you might do smaller loads or do the job several times a week instead of all at once. Give one of these alternatives a try. If it doesn't help, try another. Keep trying until you hit upon an idea that works, Dr. Maby suggests. Do this for all three tasks. Then pick three other painful chores to conquer.

other bathroom essentials. The foam tubing increases the size of the handle and makes the item easier to grasp. (Foam tubing also can be used on kitchen utensils, Nakayama says.) As for makeup, put foam tubing onto eyeliner and mascara handles for a better grip.

In the Kitchen

Conquer chaos. An efficient kitchen is a pain-free kitchen, Goodwin says. So store between eye and hip level the equipment and supplies that you regularly use. That will minimize bending, stooping, reaching, and other painful motions. Stash bread, cereal boxes, and other dry breakfast foods on a counter near the toaster and refrigerator. Hang a pegboard near your stove for cooking utensils like skillets and spatulas. Cluster dry goods, mixing bowls, and measuring tools in one spot. Plan storage so that each item can be removed without lifting or sifting through others. Store canned goods, for instance, so that the same items are lined up behind one another.

Get a go-cart. A rolling utility cart is a vital kitchen tool if you have chronic pain, Goodwin says. All the essentials for a meal can be loaded onto the cart and wheeled to the dining table, eliminating several trips to the kitchen. After a meal, dishes can be collected from the table in one trip.

Crack it open. Install a jar opener that grips lids so you can use both hands to turn jars, Nakayama suggests. Like many items, jar openers are available at most specialty housewares stores.

To open frozen foods and other bagged items, place the bag on its side and use a sharp serrated knife or scissors to open the end, Goodwin suggests. Instead of using your thumbs to open milk cartons, use the heels of your hands to push back the flanges of the spout, then use a knife to pull the spout out. Open flip-top cans with a butter knife.

Seal it shut. Many foods such as cheese are sold in resealable packages these days. But these packages actually can be torturous to close and reopen if your hands ache. If you have this problem, remove the food from its original container and store it in a way that is more convenient for you, Nakayama says. You could, for instance, simply put the cheese in a plastic sandwich bag, fold the top of the bag over, and seal it with a clothespin.

Reduce chopping pain. A food processor or onion chopper can streamline slicing and dicing foods, Hernaez says. Instead of a knife, try using a pizza wheel to cut various foods. If you must use a knife, consider getting one with an angled handle. It will put less strain on your wrist and fingers. These specialized knives are available at most housewares stores.

Spray and slide. If you use cooking pots, place the pot on the counter next to the sink, and use a spray attachment to fill the pot. Then slide the pot along the counter to the stove or slip it into a cart and wheel it over. This way you'll avoid lifting heavy pots, Goodwin says. Once the water is heated, place the food you want to cook in a frying basket and lower it into the pot. When the food is done, simply lift the frying basket out and let it drip-drain over the pot. After the pot has cooled, you can slide it back to the sink and drain it.

Maximize frugality. One-pot meals require less cleanup and can be served in the same container in which they were cooked, Nakayama says. To cut down on dishwashing, serve foods on paper plates and line pans with foil.

Mop, but don't drop. Long-handled brooms, mops, and dustpans take the strain off your back and knees, Nakayama says.

Spread Out the Load

Use larger joints to prevent strain and pain in your smaller ones, urges Denyse Hernaez, O.T., an occupational therapist at the Hospital for Special Surgery in New York City. Use the palm of your hand, for instance, instead of a fingertip to push down on spray cans. Close lids with your palm as well. To wring out a wet towel or washcloth, drape the item over a faucet and squeeze out the excess water between the palms of your hands.

In the Rest of the House

Shrink your laundry loads. Line your hamper with a plastic grocery bag, Goodwin suggests. When it is full, simply remove the bag by the handles and carry it to the washing machine. The bag will remind you to do smaller, lighter loads of laundry. Avoid overloading the bag.

Douse the dust. Keep your fingers flat and extended while dusting, Goodwin says. Switch arms to distribute the workload. A dusting mitt is worth the investment.

Can the canister. Upright vacuum cleaners require less physical energy than canister or tank models, Goodwin says. If you must use a canister vacuum, try nudging it around the room with your feet rather than pulling it with your arms. It's less stressful on your joints and muscles.

Bottle the nozzle. Aerosol spray nozzles can be difficult to use if you're in pain. Look for cleaners in easy-to-use containers or invest in an adaptor, Goodwin says. These adaptors replace the spray button with an easier-to-use pump handle that can be switched from one can to another. Spray-can adaptors are available at many housewares stores.

Take up a collection. As you clean, place in a basket any items that belong elsewhere. When you're done cleaning each room, carry the basket with you and drop the items in their appropriate places as you go about your chores, Hernaez suggests. It will help clean more efficiently and conserve energy.

To order self-help aids through the mail, write to the Rehabilitation Division of Smith and Nephew at 1 Quality Drive, Germantown, WI 53022-4422 and ask for its free consumer products catalog. Or write to the Customer Service Department of Sammons Preston at P.O. Box 5071, Bolingbrook, IL 60440-5071 and ask for its enrichments catalog.

PART TWO

Putting Your Pain to Rest

———————————

Jack Benny knew how to make people laugh. His secret weapon was simple: Mix an ounce of droll wit with a pound of truth. So, predictably, once when he was giving an acceptance speech at an awards ceremony, the comic quipped, "I don't deserve this, but I have arthritis, and I don't deserve that either."

Like Benny, we all get aches and pains we don't deserve—a toothache here, a backache there, a twinge of arthritis everywhere. And like this great jester, most of us can joke about our discomforts occasionally. But often aches and pains aren't funny. They just hurt. And just as often, the natural inclination is to blame the pains on aging and conclude that nothing can be done.

Our message here is a different one. Most of the pains that you experience actually have little to do with the process of aging. What's more, in reality there are plenty of things you can do to relieve even the most intractable discomforts well into your older years.

The next several chapters offer an in-depth look at the causes of and the treatments for some of the worst pains you're likely to face. By the end of this section, we hope you will emerge with the knowledge you need to get what you really deserve—a pain-free life.

Ankle Pain

An ankle is different from many other joints. Why? Because most of the damage that it can sustain happens suddenly. A simple misstep off a curb—and pop goes the ankle. Doctors say the number-one cause of ankle pain is sprain, where the ligaments get pulled or torn, leading to swelling, tenderness, and sometimes a bruise.

Try RICE. For the first few days after an ankle sprain, doctors recommend the RICE (rest, ice, compression, and elevation) treatment plan. But after that, RICE is not enough. You have to gently exercise a sprained ankle back to health. Exercise is important because it reduces the amount of scar tissue that develops after a sprain. Too much scar tissue, and you'll lose mobility in the ankle joint. Doctors recommend mild stretching and strengthening exercises.

Make Sure It Heals Properly

To help resolve swelling and soreness, try some gentle stretching exercises to restore flexibility in the ankle's ligaments, tendons, and muscles, suggests Kim Fagan, M.D., a sports medicine physician at the Alabama Sports Medicine and Orthopedic Center in Birmingham.

Exercise those toes. Sitting on a chair, extend your legs in front of you, about 3 inches off the floor. Focus on your toes, and try to turn them back toward you as far as you can. Hold for a few seconds. Then tip your toes forward so that they point straight out in front of you. Again, hold for a few seconds. Try 5 repetitions at first, and work up to 15 twice a day, suggests Dr. Fagan.

"This back-and-forth motion will get the muscles in the lower leg working and help dissipate any swelling," she says. "You should feel a little discomfort, but don't push to the point of pain."

Try the ankle alphabet. Have some fun and help your ankles at the same time with this toe-spelling alphabet exercise.

Slip off your shoes, and sit on a chair or the floor. Using your big toe as a pointer, rotate your ankle in the air to write the letter A. Be sure you pivot around your ankle. Don't just move your whole leg.

Continue through the alphabet. For variety, write your name in the air.

"You should feel your ankle moving slowly in different ways," says Dr. Fagan. "This stretch improves your lateral (side-to-side) and medial (inside-and-outside) movement."

Play foot tennis. Here's a sprain-recovery stretch recommended by Michael Ciccotti, M.D., an orthopedic surgeon and director of sports medicine at the Rothman Institute at Thomas Jefferson University in Philadelphia. "Try this as soon as comfort allows," he says. "Some swelling is okay."

Sit on a chair with both feet flat on the floor. Tuck a tennis ball between the arches of your feet. Gripping the ball, raise and extend your legs so that your heels are 3 to 4 inches off the floor.

Find Out What Gives

Before beginning any exercise program for ankle pain, it's important to be sure that you don't have something more serious than a sprain, such as a ruptured Achilles tendon or a fracture, says Kim Fagan, M.D., sports medicine physician at the Alabama Sports Medicine and Orthopedic Center in Birmingham. So a visit to the doctor may be in order.

"If you have a lot of tenderness right over the bone and it is extremely painful to stand, you may have a fracture," says Dr. Fagan. "Also, if there is a significant amount of swelling in the back of the ankle, it may be a problem with the Achilles tendon and not a typical sprain."

If you feel pain directly on the ankle bone, not merely an ache or tenderness on a muscle or tendon, that's another clear signal to stop exercising and see your doctor, she emphasizes.

Next, holding the ball between your feet, slowly rotate both ankles clockwise. Try 10 clockwise circles and then 10 counterclockwise circles. Remember to make the circles by rotating your ankles, not just by moving your legs and feet. Start and end your day with this stretch.

"You are restoring the range of motion to your ankle in a coordinated fashion," explains Dr. Ciccotti. "It stretches the joint capsule and the ligaments."

Table your pain. You can deliver a complete stretch from your foot all the way up your calf muscle with this exercise, recommended by Jeffrey Willson, a certified athletic trainer at K Valley Orthopedics in Kalamazoo, Michigan. Here's what to do if your ankle has been sprained.

- From a standing position, lean forward against a table with your hands palm down on the table edge and your arms straight. Stand far enough away so that you feel a moderate stretch in your calf muscles.
- Lock the leg with the sprained ankle at the knee. Slide the other leg forward, and bend it so that your knee is directly over your toes. Keep your heels on the floor.
- Press your upper body forward (don't bend at the waist) until you feel a moderate stretch in the calf muscles of your back leg. Hold that stretch for 15 to 20 seconds.
- Keeping both heels on the floor, bend your back leg until you feel a moderate stretch in your Achilles tendon. Hold that stretch for 15 to 20 seconds.
- To give your good ankle a healthy stretch, change your position and repeat the steps with your other leg.

Strengthening the Ankle

Round two of sprain recovery is returning power to the ankle's ligaments, muscles, and tendons, says Dr. Fagan. For the next three exercises, you will need something to pull on that will provide resistance. The ideal equipment is a resistance band, available at sporting goods stores. If that's not handy, a bike inner tube will do.

Dr. Fagan recommends that after you complete these exercises to give your sprained ankle a workout, repeat them with your good ankle to keep it in top shape.

Move it out and up. Sit barefoot on a chair with your aching foot directly facing the leg of a sturdy table. Loop one end of the resistance band around your foot at the base of your toes (your feet and toes should be slightly flexed). Loop the other end around the table leg about 2 inches above the floor. Keeping your heel on the floor, pull your toes back and slowly turn

No Sprain, No Pain: A Question of Balance

Lots of sprains happen because you lose your balance, stumble, and land on one of your feet at an odd angle. Here's a better-balance tip from Kim Fagan, M.D., sports medicine physician at the Alabama Sports Medicine and Orthopedic Center in Birmingham.

Strike the one-legged pose. You may snicker at the flamingo's one-legged pose, but the bird has a brain when it comes to balancing acts.

To improve your balance, try standing on one leg. Keeping your right leg slightly bent, simply lift your left leg off the floor. If you're nervous about being unsteady, put a chair in front of you for support if you wobble. After 1 minute of standing on your right leg, switch legs.

If you're feeling brave, try the one-legged stance with your eyes closed. "Keeping your eyes closed makes your body adjust without the aid of visual cues," says Dr. Fagan. It will help you achieve better balance.

Oh, in case you're wondering, according to *The Guinness Book of World Records*, in 1992 Girish Sharma of Deori, India, established the world record for standing on one leg, with a time of 55 hours and 35 minutes.

your foot outward, pulling the band taut. Repeat this five times.

Move it in and up. For the second band stretch, start with your foot in the same position as before. With your heel on the floor, slowly turn your ankle inward while flexing your toes as high as you can. Feel the resistance from the band. Try five stretches.

Pull straight. For the final strength-building exercise, start with your heel on the floor and your toes facing the table leg. This time, flex your toes straight back as far as you can. Feel the tug-of-war from the band. Try five repetitions.

Back Pain

Physical therapist Peggy Anglin, P.T., makes a living from bad backs. But more than 20 years of demonstrating the wrong moves finally caught up with her.

"I spent so much time demonstrating the wrong techniques over and over again to my patients that I became a statistic myself," says Anglin, who practices at Duke University Medical Center in Durham, North Carolina. "I was picking up a paper one morning at home, and it just hit me. I nearly fainted from the excruciating, terrifying pain."

Almost all people experience acute lower-back problems at some time in their adult lives. One of every two American adults experiences back pain every year. For people under age 45, lower-back problems rank as the top disability.

Why is back pain so common?

It's simple, sort of. The back is an amazingly complex piece of anatomical real estate. Our spines are made up of small bones called vertebrae that are stacked on top of one another like dinner plates. Sandwiched between the vertebrae are cushionlike disks. Openings in the vertebrae line up to form a long, hollow canal through which the spinal cord runs. Nerves from the spinal cord pass through small gaps between the vertebrae. When you add the dozens of back muscles, it's easy to see why backs often go blooey.

Not only is back pain widespread; it's also tough to track down. Pinpointing the cause and even the precise location of back pain often turns doctors into body detectives. "When one muscle in the back becomes inflamed or spasms, it affects a whole bunch of muscles that may structurally have nothing to do with it," says Patrick Massey, M.D., Ph.D., an internist at Alexian Brothers Medical Center in Elk Grove Village, Illinois. "Sometimes, moving your skull will affect your tailbone."

Just about the only back-pain certainty is that no one magic exercise program cures all backs. "Everybody is completely different," says Dr. Massey. "The back pain is specific to each person."

But there's hope. First, much back pain is preventable. Second, 80 to 90 percent of people with back pain recover within 6 weeks. And third, experts say that even people who have chronic back pain can often manage it—with exercise.

When Pain Strikes

Get horizontal—then get going. Rest, not exercise, is what most doctors recommend *initially* for acute back pain. "But we tell people that in order to get their circulation going, they need to be up and walking around for 45 minutes out of every 3 hours," says Brent V. Lovejoy, D.O., an occupational medicine specialist in Denver and a medical consultant to the construction industry. "Otherwise, they stiffen up like a board, and everything they do hurts."

When to See a Doctor

Here are signs it's time to see a doctor for your back pain, according to Patrick Massey, M.D., Ph.D., an internist at Alexian Brothers Medical Center in Elk Grove Village, Illinois, and a former sciatica sufferer.

- The problem persists beyond 4 days without improvement.
- You have back pain that persists after a fall or accident.
- The pain travels down your leg into the foot.

If you have any of the following symptoms, see a doctor immediately, says Dr. Massey.

- You have trouble controlling your bowels or bladder.
- You have numbness in the groin or rectal area.
- Your legs feel extremely weak.

Don't overdo a rest stop. More than 2 days' bed rest may not be helpful, according to Richard A. Deyo, M.D., D.P.H., professor in the departments of medicine and health services at the University of Washington in Seattle.

He found that back-pain sufferers who were advised to stay in bed 2 days missed 45 percent fewer days of work during the following 3 months than patients advised to rest for a full week. Muscles may weaken quickly with bed rest, and weak muscles can perpetuate an aching back.

Turn to aspirin, Advil, or Tylenol. Any over-the-counter painkiller that contains aspirin, ibuprofen (Advil), or acetaminophen (Tylenol) could ease your back pain, according to Scott Haldeman, M.D., D.C., Ph.D., associate clinical professor in the department of neurology at the University of California, Irvine, and adjunct professor at the Los Angeles Chiropractic College. But don't use painkillers before the fact. "If you know you are going to have back pain if you do something such as running, it's better not to do the activity than to mask your pain with drugs," says Dr. Haldeman.

Oh, My Achy Back

If you sometimes have back pain, you should try to make some low-stress, low-intensity aerobic exercise part of your routine. Walking, stationary biking (with upright handlebars), and swimming are healthy choices, say physical therapists. In addition, between attacks of pain, these targeted activities and exercises may bolster your back.

Chart your course. Yoga stretches, called asanas, may help relieve some back pain, says Alice Christensen, founder and executive director of the American Yoga Association in Sarasota, Florida. But be sure to get your doctor's approval before trying this or other yoga poses. With this pose, Christensen suggests, pretend that you're an ocean liner slicing through the deep blue.

- Lie on your stomach with your arms outstretched in front of you, your forehead on the floor.
- Exhale completely, then inhale as you raise your legs, arms, and head all at once, looking up. Lift yourself only as far as you can comfortably.
- Exhale and lower your body. Rest completely, then repeat two more times.

Slip into the pool. Water provides buoyancy and allows your tender muscles the chance to move freely without a lot of resistance, says Jane Sullivan-Durand, M.D., a behavioral medicine physician in Contoocook, New Hampshire. Here's a tip: Swim gentle laps for at least 10 to 12 minutes in a pool with a water temperature of at least 83°F. Warm water helps relax back muscles.

No pool? Head for a hot shower. "Try 10 minutes under a hot shower with the water beating on the affected area," says Dr. Sullivan-Durand. "Moist heat is best because dry heat from heating pads tends to increase inflammation and stiffness."

Try a pseudo-situp. Patrick Fallon, P.T., a physical therapist with the Texas Back Institute in Plano, suggests this modified situp. (Don't attempt this exercise if you are currently experiencing back pain.)

Lie on your back with your knees bent in a comfortable position and your hands on your thighs. Lift your head and shoulders off the floor slowly as you slide your fingertips to reach your knees. Hold for a count of three, and gradually ease back down. Start slowly, but aim for three sets of 10 repetitions.

Stretch like an elephant. Pretend that you're Dumbo with this back stretch offered by Meir Schneider, Ph.D., a licensed massage therapist, founder of the Center and School for Self-Healing in San Francisco, and creator of the Meir Schneider Self-Healing Method.

Stand up and bend your torso forward as far as is comfortable. Let your arms hang loosely at your sides. Next, swing your arms gently from side to side like the trunk of a contented elephant. This relieves pressure in the sacrum—the lower part of the spine—and loosens your hip and lower-back muscles. After a minute of swaying, uncurl your spine and slowly straighten to a standing position. Bring your head up last. Repeat these steps at least six times a day, says Dr. Schneider.

Enjoy a massage. Ask a friend or partner to give you a gentle rub, using the following technique, suggests Dr. Sullivan-Durand.

Five Days to a Happier Back

Although there is no one-plan-fits-all cure for back pain, Jane Sullivan-Durand, M.D., a behavioral medicine physician in Contoocook, New Hampshire, offers these general day-to-day guidelines for the first few days after the pain strikes.

Day 1: Keep your hips level. If your back feels good enough for you to drive, here are some pain-cutting tips. Place a rolled-up towel behind your lower back for support and, if you're a man, remove your wallet from your back pocket. A fat wallet makes you lopsided and can put pressure on the sciatic nerve, which could send shooting pain up your legs and back.

Day 2: Ice the pain. Frozen peas in a bag, ice cubes wrapped in a washcloth, or a chilled gel pack will restrict bloodflow to the injured spot and cut down on the chance of inflammation.

"It may be uncomfortable or even hurt at first, but tolerate the hurt until the skin feels numb," says Dr. Sullivan-Durand. "Then you know the cold has penetrated. Leaving it on for no more than 20 minutes at a time, two or three times a day or whenever the area feels hot, seems to work the best."

Using either both thumbs or the heels of both hands, your friend or partner should rub up from the center of your spine, starting at the bottom of the back and stopping just below the shoulder blades. Then your friend or partner should start over again at the bottom. Massage stimulates the circulation of blood and lymphatic fluid (which tends to accumulate around an injury site). This kind of massage reduces swelling and promotes healing, says Dr. Sullivan-Durand.

Day 3: Turn to massage. When you feel that the ache is more tolerable, ask your spouse or a friend to lend you a hand. "A muscle that is tight can usually be manually softened and released through massage," Dr. Sullivan-Durand says. "Have them run their fingers along the sore area and feel the spasm. Ask them to take their thumbs or the heels of their hands and stroke that area as deeply as possible without causing any discomfort. Don't squeeze the area."

Day 4: Start stretching. Start the morning with this stretch. Lie on your back on the floor or bed, your feet flat and your knees bent. Use both hands to bring your left knee to your chest. Hold for 10 seconds. Repeat with your right knee. Repeat once more, this time bringing both knees up at once.

This exercise helps to loosen your lower-back muscles and can become part of your daily routine even after the back pain subsides, Dr. Sullivan-Durand says.

Day 5: See a doctor or take a walk. This is judgment day. If your back still isn't up to par, see a doctor, advises Dr. Sullivan-Durand. If you feel better, put on your sneakers and do a 30-minute steady walk on level ground or on a treadmill.

How to Prevent a Back Attack

There are no guarantees. But doctors and physical therapists agree that you can reduce the chance of getting back pain. Here's how.

- Avoid lifting while twisting, bending forward, or reaching.
- Bend at the knees, not at the waist, when lifting.
- Lose excess weight, especially in the abdomen.

- Improve your posture. Keep your natural back curves in alignment by lifting your breastbone and maintaining a slight hollow in your lower back.
- Don't sleep on your stomach. Lie on your side with your knees bent or on your back with a small pillow under your knees.
- Make exercise part of your daily routine. Take walks, swim, and tone up your abdominal and back muscles through exercises. Stay flexible.

The Back-Pain Sufferer's Guide to Gardening, Golf, and Love

Having back pain doesn't mean that you must give up doing the things you love. But you may have to customize your technique and develop some pain-avoidance strategies. Physical therapists offer these tips to help you keep enjoying your hobbies, sports, and other leisure activities.

Dig

There are enough twists in gardening and yard work to make Chubby Checker jealous. To avoid pain while working, keep these thoughts in mind.

Pace yourself. If you're a weekend gardener who tries to get everything done on Saturday, you might want to be a little kinder to your back. "People tend to go from doing nothing during the week to gardening for 4 hours or more on the weekend," says Wendy Woods, P.T., a physical therapist at K Valley Orthopedics in Kalamazoo, Michigan. Take a break every half-hour, she says.

When hoeing, use short motions. The smaller the chopping motions, the less strain on your back muscles, says Anglin. "When you're using a hoe, you don't need to swing your arms in wide, big motions," she says. "With

Don't Buy Back Pain at the Supermarket

Many back injuries are caused by lifting something that's too heavy at a tough angle, says Jane Sullivan-Durand, M.D., a behavioral medicine physician from Contoocook, New Hampshire. Here's her pain-free way to load groceries into your car.

- Position the grocery cart next to your open trunk or car door.
- Bend your knees slightly, keeping your back straight.
- Lift a bag from the cart, using both hands underneath it, then bring it close to your body, still holding it at the bottom.
- To place a bag in the car, bend your knees first, keeping your back as straight as possible. Don't bend from the waist or overextend your arms when putting the bag into your trunk or backseat. Remember to keep your arms slightly bent.

"Never use only your arms and upper back to lift groceries," she says. "That puts strain on your lower and middle back."

hoes, brooms, or mops, keep your upper arms close to your sides. Use your leg muscles for power, not your back."

Weed with your knees. Get up close to those wicked weeds by getting down on your hands and knees, says Anglin. "Crawling around on your hands and knees is a fine position for the back," she says. "It's much better than bending over and rounding your back to pull weeds. That position puts a lot of stress on your lower back."

Stop rake ache. Woods offers this leaf-raking tip for autumn weekends. When you're raking, be sure to stand really upright. Use your knees and hips so that the power of your legs can help your arms pull the leaves. And take stretch breaks every 15 minutes.

Swing

Golf, because it involves so much twisting, can sometimes cause back pain. "We get a lot of golfers here at the center," says Woods. "They want to keep golfing and don't want to stop at any cost." Try these ideas to deal with hacker's back.

Slow down. In general, Woods recommends that golfers with bum backs slow down their strokes to reduce stress on the lower back. Remember the wisdom of Bobby Jones, the biggest name in golf during the 1920s: A golf club cannot be swung too slowly.

Shorten your swing. A long backswing is not just bad golf strategy; it's also bad back medicine. Wendy Woods says that shortening your backswing by not pulling back so far with the club reduces twisting and the strain on your back.

Meet the tee. When it's time to tee up the ball or pull it out of the cup, posture is key, says Woods. "Don't bend from the back. Try to bend at the knees, keep your back in a neutral position, and slowly lower yourself down to put the ball on the tee or take it out of the hole."

Get symmetrical. If you carry your bag, be sure to use a strap that goes over both shoulders. That way, you distribute the weight evenly, which may prevent some back problems caused by habitual overuse of one side of the back.

Cuddle

Your hormones scream yes; your back says no way. You can win this battle by practicing safe sex for backs, say physical therapists. The most important things are to keep the spine aligned properly and to use positions that don't require the partner with back pain to be active or bear weight, says Anglin. Try these back-safe positions.

Spoon your mate. In this position, both partners lie on their sides with their knees bent and the man behind the woman. Nobody bears any body weight, Woods says.

Try a pillow prop. Here, the partner with the bad back lies on his back, using pillows to support the neck and lower back if necessary. This provides a stabler position for the back during sex, says Woods. If the man has a bad back, his partner should straddle him with her knees bent while supporting her upper-body weight with her arms. If it's the woman who has a bad back, her partner should support himself with his arms and knees so that little weight falls on her.

Head for the hot tub. Let buoyancy and the warm, massaging bubbles of a hot tub keep both of you in the mood, says Woods. She recommends that the man sit in the tub with the woman sitting on his thighs and facing him. This position will work if either the man or the woman has a bad back, she notes. "The key here is to not make twisting motions," Woods adds.

Bursitis and Tendinitis

Think of a garden hose bulging with water in one spot. That's bursitis. Now picture a clothesline stretched beyond its comfortable limits. That's tendinitis.

Every day, our bodies rely on dozens of bursae and taut tendons to keep our muscles and joints moving smoothly. Bursae are sacs or saclike cavities filled with lubricating fluid and sandwiched in where muscles or tendons pass over bony places. Tendons are taffylike cords that attach muscles to bones.

Problems develop from overuse. Sometimes the soreness and stiffness is caused by that nonstop weekend tennis tournament. And sometimes it's an occupational hazard of living, a result of years of wear and tear—from swinging a golf club, raking leaves, or just reaching for the pickle jar on the top shelf. As we get older, our bursae and tendons often become more vulnerable.

Shoulders are choice spots for flare-ups, but both bursitis and tendinitis can develop in the knees, hips, and elbows as well. It can be difficult to tell whether you have bursitis, tendinitis, or both. The signs and symptoms can be similar, including pain and irritation when you move and when you're trying to sleep. Bursitis may come with more noticeable inflammation and can seem to be more severe. If pain or inflammation is persistent for more than 2 to 3 days, you should see a doctor for an accurate diagnosis.

Bursitis and tendinitis are very seldom life-threatening, says John Cianca, M.D., assistant professor of physical medicine and rehabilitation and director of the sports and human performance medicine program at Baylor College of Medicine in Houston. He adds, however, that some cases are more serious than others and may require surgical correction. Chronic joint instability and a torn rotator cuff tendon are such examples.

Dealing With the Pain

Give it a rest. This might sound obvious, but because bursitis and tendinitis are often triggered by using a body part in a way that it's not used to, rest is one of the first steps on the road to recovery. "Complete rest is necessary in order for the pain to subside," says Keith Jones, head trainer for the Houston Rockets basketball team. Whatever activity triggered the bout of bursitis or tendinitis, avoid it for 3 to 6 weeks, if possible. Even multimillion-dollar athletes take a break when they have bursitis and tendinitis—you should, too.

Try some ice. In addition to rest, Jones recommends putting ice wrapped in a thin towel on the area that ails you. "If you suffer from bursitis or tendinitis, make sure you apply ice to the sore area for 20 minutes at least three times per day," says Jones. "The combination of the rest and the ice should pay noticeable dividends within days."

Don't use heat. If you're suffering from bursitis or tendinitis, resist the urge to apply a heating pad to the affected joint, says William Pesanelli, physical therapist and the director of Boston University's rehabilitation services. "It's like pouring lighter fluid on an already existing fire," he cautions. "If you're suffering from bursitis or tendinitis, the tissues in the sore area are already inflamed and will feel warmer to touch than the rest of your body, so adding heat will only make matters worse." Instead, you'll find more relief by using ice until the inflammation is gone.

Babying Bursitis

Once the pain and swelling subside, you should do some mild stretching exercises, says Dan Hamner, M.D., a physiatrist and sports medicine specialist in New York City.

"With bursitis, you have to be careful and hold back a bit on activity," he says. "But if you totally rest an extremity for too long, you'll lose strength and range of motion. This is particularly true for the shoulder."

Try some shoulder soothers. For shoulder bursitis, Dr. Hamner offers the following easy movements to restore range of motion and keep the swelling down. Before all of these exercises, he recommends doing 5 minutes of ice treatment (simply wrap some ice in a towel and hold it on the painful area). He also suggests controlled, slow movements for best results.

- Stand and bend forward at the waist at a 45-degree angle.
- Let both arms hang loosely straight down, parallel to your legs, and bend your knees slightly to keep pressure off your back.
- Move one arm clockwise in a small circle; in 10 rotations, increase the size of the circle from about 1 foot to about 3 feet in diameter, allowing your entire arm, from your shoulder to your hand, to rotate.

- Wind down in another 10 rotations back to the smallest circle.
- Then try the rotations counterclockwise, using the same arm movement.
- Repeat the sequence on the other side. Try this exercise three to five times a day.

For variety—and only if your shoulders can tolerate it—try this exercise with a 1- or 2-pound weight in each hand, says Dr. Hamner.

Remember how those toy soldiers from the movie *Babes in Toyland* swung their arms dramatically back and forth? Well, that kind of arm movement can help beat bursitis, says Dr. Hamner. Here's how to do it.

- Stand with your feet shoulder-width apart and your arms at your sides.
- Raise your injured arm as if you were raising your hand in class. Keep your elbow locked. Stop about 10 degrees short of vertical, with the palm of your hand facing forward.
- At the same time, extend your other arm, with your elbow locked and the palm of your hand facing your leg, behind you about 10 degrees. Hold this stretch for 1 to 2 seconds.
- In a controlled manner, gently swing your injured arm down and back and your other arm forward and up. Each arm should mirror the previous position of the opposite arm.
- Repeat 10 times, alternating arms.

"Doing these motions slowly should help bring relief to the bursae," says Dr. Hamner.

Help your hips. The hips are another common spot for bursitis, says Dr. Hamner. Here's a stretch to ease the pain. Ice the spot for 5 minutes before giving this a try.

- Lie flat on your back with your knees bent and your feet flat on the floor.
- Using your abdominal and quadriceps (front of thigh) muscles, and your hands if you need to, raise your legs.
- In a slow, controlled movement, bring your knees toward your chest as far as you can.
- Hold the stretch for 2 to 3 seconds.
- Relax and slowly lower your legs back to the original position.
- Repeat this stretch 10 times.

Taming Tendinitis

Tendons that have been inflamed prefer gentle massages and some stretches to return to full flexibility, says Dr. Cianca. Once full flexibility is restored and the pain is alleviated, strengthening exercises should be added.

Drop your heels to ease your Achilles. The Achilles tendon, the thick band that attaches your calf muscles to your heel bone, often becomes irritated. According to doctors, these exercises will help ease the pain and repair the tendon.

The first exercise, a stair stretch, is fairly vigorous, but the Achilles is a tough, long tendon, and it takes a fair amount of effort to overcome tightness, according to Dr. Cianca.

- Stand on a step with your heels hanging over the edge. To bolster your balance, hold the railing.
- Gradually drop your heels until you feel a stretch, but not pain. Try to hold the stretch for 20 to 30 seconds.
- Then step off and let your feet rest on the floor in a neutral position. Repeat this exercise two more times, says Dr. Cianca.

Write with your feet. Here's an exercise that gives your Achilles tendon a little bit of stretch but doesn't over-stretch it.

- Sit in a hot tub or whirlpool or a bathtub with your feet under the stream of warm water from the faucet.
- Pretend to write the letters of the alphabet with your feet. Be sure to include letters that involve a lot of pointing and flexing, recommends Dr. Hamner. If making letters doesn't appeal to you, try doing foot circles—25 one way and 25 the other. (You can do the same exercises while seated.)

Pick a pair of elbow aids. For elbow tendinitis relief, you'll need support from a sturdy tabletop, suggests Carl Fried, P.T., a physical therapist at K Valley Orthopedics in Kalamazoo, Michigan.

- Sit facing the long end of a narrow table.
- Stretch the painful arm across to the far side of the table so that your wrist hangs completely over the edge and your fingers are extended. Keep your arm straight, with your elbow locked and your palm facing down.
- Grasp the back of that hand with your other hand and slowly try to bend the wrist down as far as possible.
- Hold for 10 seconds and then release.
- Repeat these steps up to 10 times twice a day.

Or try a variation on this exercise. Head for the pantry and grab a can that fits your grip. Put your arm in the same position along the edge of the tabletop—palm down and wrist over the edge—but hold the can in your hand. Gently move your wrist up and down 25 times. Pause for a few seconds, then do 25 more. Try this twice a day, says Fried.

Try a shoulder solution. A door frame can be a true ally against shoulder tendinitis, either as a good preventive measure or whenever pain strikes, says Dr. Hamner. He recommends doing at least four stretches twice a day.

- Step inside a door opening.
- Place your palms and forearms flat on the jamb on each side of the door frame, your hands slightly above shoulder level.
- Gently lean forward through the doorway while your lower arms bear the weight. You should feel a stretch in both shoulders.
- Hold the stretch for at least 6 seconds.

Knead your knees. To relieve tendinitis in your knees, Dr. Hamner recommends doing what he calls cross-friction finger massage.

- Sit in a chair.
- If your right knee is red and swollen, cup your right hand across the front of that knee so that your index finger is on top of the painful area and lying across the tendon running down the front of the knee.
- Place your middle finger on top of your index finger.
- Press down and gently massage the painful spot, working your fingers firmly for 5 to 7 minutes. This could be painful at first, but it should ease up. If your fingers get tired, knead the spot with your thumb.

Carpal Tunnel Syndrome

Picture New York City's Lincoln Tunnel during Friday-afternoon rush hour. Thousands of cars, trucks, and buses stream into the tunnel. Horns sound and tempers flare as congestion builds and traffic comes to a halt. Well, some people have a similar tunnel of torment in their hands and wrists.

Your carpal tunnel is a passageway of bone and ligament in your wrist. The traffic through it consists of nine tendons and the median nerve, the major nerve between your arm and your fingers. If the tendons in the tunnel become inflamed or fill with fluid, they can swell, pinching the median nerve. This often causes pain, tingling, and numbness in the fingers.

Often, carpal tunnel syndrome (CTS) is caused by repetitive strain injury, which is the result of over-and-over-again wrist or finger motion, especially if it's combined with gripping vibrating tools or using instruments that put pressure at the base of the palm. People who type, sew, hammer, or paint for many hours every day often get the tendon swelling that causes the nerve pain.

You may experience tingling, numbness, or pain in the hand and fingers, especially in the thumb and first two fingers. The more you use your hand, the more it will hurt. As the condition progresses, your hand can become so weak that you can't even grip a glass. For severe cases like this, a doctor may recommend surgery to relieve pressure on the entrapped nerve.

Try These First

You may be able to get relief and reduce inflammation right away with simple measures like splinting your wrist in a neutral position and altering your activity. Here are other ways to get relief.

Pack on an ice pack. You may find that the pain lessens when you put an ice pack on your wrist, according to Steven Barrer Jr., M.D., a clinical assistant professor of neurosurgery at the Medical College of Pennsylvania in Philadelphia, who has written numerous articles on CTS. "If you use an ice pack (a bag of frozen vegetables works fine), wrap it in a dish towel and hold it between your wrists for 10 to 15 minutes, then remove it for about the same amount of time, and repeat. This will prevent a freeze burn."

Or warm your wrists with a heating pad. Others find relief by holding a heating pad or warm compress between their wrists to relax muscles, adds Dr. Barrer. "The best thing to do is try both and see what works for you."

Get a boost with vitamin B₆. This nutrient seems to help relieve the symptoms of CTS, says Jill Stansbury, N.D., assistant professor of botanical medicine and chair of the botanical medicine department at the National College of Naturopathic Medicine in Portland, Oregon. It works best on mild to moderate cases, says Thomas Kruzel, N.D., a naturopathic doctor in Portland, Oregon. To end the tingling, take 50 milligrams of B_6 each day, he suggests, and give it time to work. It usually takes 12 weeks to get the full benefit. You can boost the healing power of B_6 by taking at least 10 milligrams of riboflavin along with it, says Dr. Kruzel.

Look to an herb with nerve. Widely known for its ability to treat depression, St. John's wort also helps nerves recover when they are damaged, inflamed, or strained, says Dr. Stansbury. Its sedative effect helps to reduce pain, while its anti-inflammatory activity can help shrink swollen tendons. Don't expect the kind of quick pain relief that comes from popping a pharmaceutical like aspirin or ibuprofen, though; St. John's wort typically takes a few weeks to start working. Start out with 150 to 250 milligrams of extract standardized to 0.3 percent hypericin three times a day, says Dr. Stansbury. You should start to see some improvement in about 2 weeks. If you don't, take a little more, she says—300 to 400 milligrams three times a day.

While St. John's wort is generally very safe, pregnant women should not take it without a doctor's okay.

Add some flaxseed oil. You can soothe inflamed nerve and tissues with flaxseed oil, a supplement rich in omega-3 essential fatty acids, says Ellen Potthoff, D.C., N.D., a chiropractor and naturopathic doctor in Pleasant Hill, California. You should feel better in 2 to 4 weeks if you take 1 tablespoon of flaxseed oil every day, she says.

Experience the power of turmeric. This herb contains a powerful anti-inflammatory chemical called curcumin. The effect of turmeric has been compared with that of cortisone, the pharmaceutical sometimes used to treat CTS. Although turmeric's pain-fighting power is not as strong as cortisone's, the herb is a lot easier on your system, says Dr. Kruzel. He gives people with CTS 250 to 500 milligrams of curcumin a day. Keep taking this dose

Punching Your Way out of Carpal Tunnel

Marketing director Marcia Miller dodged hand surgery for carpal tunnel syndrome by throwing punches with former world middleweight contender Michael Olajide Jr.

Years of repetitive computer keyboard work had caught up with her, causing loss of most of the movement in her right hand and some in her left. Since aspirin and other painkillers couldn't ease the throbbing, doctors recommended hand surgery to open up the carpal tunnel. But she searched for a more natural alternative.

Dan Hamner, M.D., a physiatrist and sports medicine specialist in New York City, introduced Miller to Aerobox. This highly aerobic program incorporates the jabs, upper-

until the inflammation has been reduced, he advises, then take half that dose for 1 to 2 weeks until your symptoms are gone. If the symptoms return, repeat with the high dose, and return to the lower dose again after they improve.

Do not use turmeric supplements without talking to your doctor, especially if you are pregnant.

Pain-Fighting Toys and Games

Severe cases of carpal tunnel syndrome cannot be healed by exercise, and doctors caution that you should stop any wrist or finger exercise if there is constant pain or total numbness. But moderate CTS can be treated cuts, hooks, head bobs, and body weaves of a boxing match without actual hitting.

Under Dr. Hamner's medical supervision and with the benefit of Olajide's boxing expertise, Miller says that her wrist became pain-free within a few months.

"With this type of shadow boxing, you are not hitting anyone, so you don't hurt your muscles or tendons," says Olajide. "Marcia gained both physical and psychological benefits from Aerobox."

Miller cites two major benefits of this exercise program. "I solved the problems with my hands and also learned more about fitness than I ever thought I would in my life," she says. "It puts you in a frame of mind that you can do anything if you set your mind to it."

with gentle exercises. The trick is to strengthen and flex the tendons and stimulate the movement of fluid out of the crowded tunnel, thus taking pressure off the median nerve.

"In carpal tunnel syndrome, it is important to have some wrist extension, wrist flexion, and side-to-side movement," says Dan Hamner, M.D., a physiatrist and sports medicine specialist in New York City. He offers these gentle—even playful—exercises.

Do the Slinky shimmy. Remember that coiled toy from your childhood? It can be an exercise tool for today, says Dr. Hamner. Simply cradle the ends in the open palms of both hands and gently move your wrists up and down as you flop the Slinky from hand to hand.

Deal yourself a great hand. The simple act of card shuffling is an ideal exercise to work the wrist muscles from side to side. When your bridge club meets, volunteer to be the steady dealer.

Do the yo-yo. The up-and-down glide of a yo-yo is a great exercise to flex and extend the wrists, says Dr. Hamner. Advanced yo-yo performers can try the cradle and walk-the-dog moves.

Gentle and Varied Exercises to Quiet the Carpal

After your symptoms are under control, exercise can help prevent the return of carpal tunnel pain. The key is to use gentle strengthening movements and to vary the motions, say doctors and physical therapists. Here are a few simple exercises that you can do while watching television or even relaxing in a bathtub.

Mimic a mime. For this wrist exercise, stand facing a wall. Extend your arms out at shoulder level directly in front of you, your palms facing the wall. Without touching the wall, pretend that you are a mime trying to find an exit from a box. Slowly move your palms and shoulders up as you reach for the imaginary ceiling, says Dr. Hamner.

Try pretend window washing. While standing or sitting, extend your arms in front of you and gently move your hands clockwise as if you were rubbing smudges off a window. Then change directions and move counterclockwise, says Dr. Hamner.

Offer some high-pressure prayer. Put your hands together as though to pray, then push the palms against each other. This helps to stretch the wrist muscles, says Susan Isernhagen, P.T., a physical therapist and director of Isernhagen Work Systems in Duluth, Minnesota. Hold the pressure for a count of five and relax. As a variation, keep your fingertips touching as you move your palms apart.

Turn to tennis balls. There's no need for a racquet or net for this strengthening exercise, offered by Dr. Hamner. Holding a tennis ball in each hand, simply extend your arms straight out in front of you, palms up. Squeeze the balls, then relax. Do this 10 times, shake out your hands, and repeat.

Reach for new heights. Here is an exercise to get the fluid out of your wrists and fight the numbness, tingling, and jabbing pain it causes by pressing against the median nerve, says Dr. Hamner.

While watching television in your favorite chair, rest your hands and elbows on top of the backrest so that your hands are behind your head—and, most important, above the level of your heart. Hold that pose during an entire commercial, and gradually build your way up to a half-hour sitcom.

A Keyboard Survival Guide

Hours at the computer keyboard are a common cause of carpal crisis. You can avoid the shooting pain through your hand and wrist by using proper computer poses and office exercises, say doctors.

"We often put ourselves in a head-forward, limb-forward posture at a computer keyboard, and that puts strain on the neck, shoulders, elbows, arms, wrists, and fingers," says Robert Markison, M.D., a hand surgeon and associate clinical professor of surgery at the University of California, San Francisco. He offers this fight-back survival guide.

- Maintain proper posture. Keep your head resting on the center between your shoulders, and avoid leaning forward.

- Avoid extreme wrist positions by keeping your wrists almost straight on the keyboard, not below it or arched upward.
- When typing, move your little fingers over to reach the keys on the edges to type the letters Q, A, and Z and the punctuation symbols. Avoid straining your tendons by stretching the little finger out.
- Don't pound the keyboard like a jackhammer. Try a kinder, gentler touch.
- Alternate tapping the space bar with your right and left thumbs to avoid overusing one thumb.
- Every 30 minutes or so, stop typing or working the mouse, and stand up and stretch.

Cold Sores

A tingling sensation outside your mouth or above your lips is usually the telltale sign. Within 2 to 3 days, a painful, fluid-filled blister appears. It swells, ruptures, and oozes fluid that forms a yellow crust. Eventually, it peels off and reveals new skin underneath. The blister usually lasts 7 to 10 days, but while it's in full view, you may be tempted to go into hiding or cover your mouth with your hands until the unsightly sore disappears.

What causes cold sores, commonly called fever blisters, is herpes simplex virus type 1 (HSV-1). About 90 percent of all people are infected with this virus, and if you get a sore once, you can be pretty sure that you'll get one again. If you change your diet and take some other natural measures against these sores, however, you might be able to shorten the time that they stay on your mouth and lips.

To prevent cold sores, some naturopathic doctors advise that you eat more foods that are high in the amino acid lysine, such as yogurt, chicken, fish, and vegetables. At the same time, they say, you should cut back on foods that are high in arginine, another amino acid. The foods to avoid include chocolate, nuts, seeds, and gelatin.

For Fast Relief

Drop a tannic bomb. If applied soon enough, over-the-counter drops (such as Zilactin-L) that contain tannic acid can prevent a cold sore from forming or, at the very least, help to reduce its size, says Brad Rodu, D.D.S., professor in the department of pathology at the University of Alabama School of Medicine in Birmingham.

The key is to start using the drops as soon as your lip begins tingling. That's an early-warning sign that a cold sore may appear in the next 4 to 12 hours, Dr. Rodu says. Reapply the drops every hour while you feel the tingling. It will help keep the sore small.

Try tea. Like some over-the-counter (OTC) drops, non-herbal tea, too, contains tannic acid. The OTC medications are more effective, but you may want to try putting a wet tea bag on the sore for a few minutes every hour to provide temporary relief until you can get to the drugstore, Dr. Rodu says.

Natural Remedies

Heal them with lysine. This amino acid inhibits the replication of herpes simplex. During an outbreak, take 3,000 milligrams of lysine daily until the lesions go away. Otherwise, at the first sign of symptoms, take 500 to 1,500 milligrams daily, says Jennifer Brett, N.D., a naturopathic doctor at the Wilton Naturopathic Center in Stratford, Connecticut. Continue with that dosage until symptoms disappear.

Zap 'em with vitamin C and bioflavonoids. These supplements boost your immune system so the blisters will heal faster, says Dr. Brett. To help heal existing sores, she recommends taking 3,000 milligrams of vitamin C daily in divided doses and 1,000 milligrams daily of quercetin, a commonly used bioflavonoid. To prevent cold sores, take 1,000 milligrams of vitamin C with bioflavonoids daily, Dr. Brett advises.

Zinc 'em, too. Upping your intake of zinc can also reduce the frequency, duration, and severity of cold sore outbreaks. During an outbreak, take 50 milligrams a day of zinc in divided doses with food, says Michael Traub, N.D., a naturopathic doctor and director of the integrated residency program at North Hawaii Community Hospital in Kamuela. As a preventive, take 20 milligrams a day. Also, since zinc supplementation can lead to copper deficiency, you should take 1 to 2 milligrams of copper for every 25 milligrams of zinc you take, says Dr. Traub. Don't exceed 2 milligrams of copper daily, however.

Reach for antiviral herbs. Echinacea and St. John's wort can also speed healing, lessen the severity, and shorten the duration of cold sores, says Dr. Traub. Echinacea strengthens the immune system. Dr. Traub recommends taking one 300-milligram capsule of echinacea four times a day during a cold sore outbreak. For prevention, take one 300-milligram capsule daily during times of stress or as soon as you feel a cold sore coming on, he says.

St. John's wort has strong antiviral properties, so it may help to prevent the herpesvirus from replicating. During a cold sore outbreak, take one 300-milligram capsule of St. John's wort daily, says Dr. Traub. Buy the standardized extract that contains 0.3 percent hypericin.

Give it a frosty reception. You may be able to lessen the severity of an outbreak, says Dr. Rodu, if you put ice on your lip at the first sign of tingling. That may slow the growth of the virus that causes cold sores. Wrap an ice cube in a towel and apply it to the affected spot for 5 to 10 minutes, repeating about once an hour.

Colds and Flu

With more than 200 cold viruses floating around and a new strain of flu just waiting to claim its next victims each year, it seems almost impossible *not* to get sick. While scientists are currently working on high-tech ways to stop these viruses from spreading, the following are some ways to cut down your risk—or at least reduce the time you spend suffering.

If these and other remedies don't have an effect, however, you may have to be on guard for other kinds of infection. Be sure to see your doctor if your cold does not improve within 14 days or if you have green or yellow phlegm. And check with your doctor if you have trouble breathing or if your temperature tops 102°F.

Feel Better Faster

Drink vitamin C–rich juice. Orange, tomato, grapefruit, or pineapple juice can help you get over a cold—but you need to drink at least five glasses a day. "Studies show it takes that much vitamin C (about 500 milligrams) to reduce sneezes and coughs in cold sufferers," says Jeffrey Jahre, M.D., clinical assistant professor of medicine at Temple University School of Medicine in Philadelphia and chief of the Infectious Diseases Section at St. Luke's Medical Center in Bethlehem, Pennsylvania. If that amount seems like a bit much to swallow, you can take vitamin C supplements. But don't go overboard. Larger doses of vitamin C can cause stomach upset in some people.

Serve a steamy bowl of comfort. Any hot liquid helps cut through congestion, but chicken soup is probably best of all, according to Frederick Ruben, M.D., professor of medicine at the University of Pittsburgh and spokesperson for the American Lung Association. No study has shown *why* chicken soup seems to work so well, but it's certain that the soup is protein rich, tasty, and a comforting way to get nutrients if you're not up to eating. "People who wouldn't drink hot water will readily eat chicken soup," says Dr. Ruben.

Don't bother with antihistamines. Over-the-counter cold medicines that contain antihistamines do little more than make you sleepy. "New findings show that histamine is not produced when you have a cold," says Dr. Ruben, so the drugs designed to fight it won't help.

By all means, feed your flu. You need vitamins and minerals to mount an effective defense against the flu bug, says Herbert Patrick, M.D., assistant professor of medicine and medical director of the respiratory care department at Jefferson Medical College of Thomas Jefferson University in Philadelphia. Aim for well-balanced meals, or at least try some bland fruit such as applesauce or mashed bananas.

Beware of fluid flu remedies. Combination cold/flu liquid remedies can contain as much as 40 percent alcohol. "That's equal to the amount in a shot of liquor," says Dr. Ruben. Alcohol can depress your immune system and also dry out your mucous membranes, so you should avoid it when you have the flu, he says.

Natural Relief

These nutritional supplements can help speed your recovery.

Look to powerful herbs. Echinacea and goldenseal, taken in combination, are top cold and flu fighters among medicinal herbal supplements, says Kristy Fassler, N.D., a naturopathic doctor in Portsmouth, New Hampshire.

When symptoms strike, take 300 milligrams of each of these herbs every 2 to 4 hours for the first 2 to 3 days, says Dr. Fassler. Continue with the same dosage of each three times a day until symptoms disappear.

Dig a root from the Orient. For thousands of years in China, the herb that has been used to enhance immunity is astragalus root. This potent herb also may help boost levels of interferon, one of your body's virus fighters, says Chris Meletis, N.D., professor of natural pharmacology at the National College of Naturopathic Medicine in Portland, Oregon. A heightened level of interferon can help prevent or shorten the duration of colds and flu.

To stamp out a cold or flu in its earliest stages, take one 500-milligram capsule of astragalus four times a day until symptoms disappear, says Dr. Meletis. Then take one capsule twice a day for 7 days to prevent a relapse.

Call on a dynamic duo. It's a good idea to stock your medicine cabinet with vitamin A and beta-carotene supplements, say Dr. Fassler and Dr. Meletis. These nutrients help you fight back fast, before the virus takes up residence and multiplies in your body.

As soon as you notice cold or flu symptoms, take 100,000 international units (IU) of vitamin A daily for 3

Preparing for Quicker Relief

In one study, researchers found that moderate exercise can help reduce the number of days that you experience symptoms once you get a cold or the flu. In the study, conducted at Loma Linda University's department of health science in California, researchers divided 50 overweight, sedentary women, ages 25 to 45, into two groups. For 15 weeks, one group walked briskly for 45 minutes 5 days a week. The women in the other group went about their normal routine.

During those weeks, researchers discovered that the exercise group had half as many days with cold symptoms as the nonexercisers. And when the scientists did blood tests, they found that the gladiators of the immune system, called natural killer cells, were more active in the exercise group. Since these killer cells help people fight off colds more quickly, their prevalence helps to explain why the exercise group had more resistance. Researchers concluded that the steady exercise provided preventive power.

So if you want to be less miserable with cold symptoms, start walking, riding, swimming, dancing, or doing any other kind of heart-pumping activity before the cold season descends on your neighborhood.

days, says Dr. Fassler, then reduce the dosage to 25,000 IU for 1 week or until symptoms disappear. She cautions, however, that these are very high doses, and you need to check with your doctor before taking this much.

Vitamin A's precursor, beta-carotene, is brimming with antioxidant power and antiviral properties. "Beta-carotene also protects you from viruses by enhancing mucous membrane secretions. By producing the secretions, the beta-carotene prevents the virus from setting up housekeeping in your body," says Thomas Kruzel, N.D., a naturopathic doctor in Portland, Oregon. If you feel a cold or the flu coming on, take 100,000 IU of beta-carotene for 10 to 14 days, says Dr. Kruzel, then cut the dosage to 50,000 IU a day to prevent future respiratory infections.

Add zinc to your diet. Of all the trace minerals found in multivitamins, zinc is probably the most important for keeping your immunity strong. A lack of zinc can increase your risk of catching a cold, the flu, or another upper respiratory infection. While it's best to get zinc from foods, you can get what you need from supplements. Be careful not to take too much—doctors recommend no more than 15 milligrams a day. If you check with your physician, you can take 30 milligrams a day with food for 7 to 10 days, but don't take more unless you have your doctor's consent.

Zinc gluconate in lozenge form has been found to shorten the duration of cold symptoms. In a study, participants who sucked on one zinc gluconate lozenge (containing about 13 milligrams of zinc) every 2 hours while awake got rid of their coughs, nasal congestion, sore throat, and headaches 3 to 4 days sooner than those who didn't get any supplementation. After checking with your doctor, you can take the lozenges to help shake off these symptoms. Don't take them for longer than 1 week, cautions Dr. Meletis, because they can weaken your immune system.

Effortless Remedies

For some people with the all-too-common cold, a modest workout might be just the thing to kick the germs. But if the problem is the flu, exercise might do as much harm as good. When can you hit the trail, and when should you hit the hay? Do a quick symptom check, suggests William A. Primos Jr., M.D., who practices primary-care sports medicine in Charlotte, North Carolina. If your symptoms are above the neck, such as a stuffy or runny nose or a sore throat, exercising is probably all right, advises Dr. Primos. But start at half speed, he cautions. If after 10 minutes you feel okay, you can increase the intensity and finish your workout. But if you feel horrible after 10 minutes, stop.

When your symptoms are below the neck, avoid exercise completely, recommends Dr. Primos. Some common symptoms that fall into this category are muscle aches, a hacking cough, a fever of 100°F or higher, chills, diarrhea, or vomiting. Many of these are indicators of the flu, and if you work out in this condition, you're likely to feel even weaker and certainly become dehydrated. If after 5 or 6 days your symptoms haven't improved or have worsened, you should see a doctor.

Whether you have a cold or flu, though, you can try some modest tactics to give you relief from symptoms. Here are some ways to put healing into motion, even if you're feeling more like lounging than doing lunges.

Practice acupressure. To help clear up a headache, use the thumb and forefinger of one hand to press and hold the top of the first joint below your thumbnail on the other hand, says Mary Muryn, a certified teacher of polarity (energy healing) and reflexology (a type of acupressure that focuses on the hands and feet) in Westport, Connecticut. "But never press for more than 5 minutes," she advises, since you can actually make your headache worse if you lean on that spot too long.

Nudge your nostrils. An acupressure technique can help relieve a clogged nose, says Michael Reed Gach, Ph.D., director of the Acupressure Institute in Berkeley, California. Place the tips of your middle and index fingers on either side of your nostrils, directly under your cheekbones. Gently press each side of your nostrils, applying pressure upward and inward while your index fingers push the area alongside your middle fingers. Hold for 2 minutes.

Press the eye area. There's another pair of acupressure points to know about, especially if you're suffering from a stuffy nose. Place your index fingers directly underneath each cheekbone again, but this time they should be under the center of each eye rather than near the nostrils. Gently press and hold for 2 minutes.

Toe, toe, toe your throat. There's an acupressure point on your big toe that can help relieve sore throat pain, according to Muryn. The point is on the underside of each toe—the area underneath where the toe curls. To reach that area, lift your foot to the opposite knee and press the underside of your big toe with your thumb, or use both thumbs for extra pressure. "You need a good deal of pressure so you really feel it," says Muryn, but don't press so hard that you're in pain. If it's hard to get the pressure in that point, you can use the eraser end of a pencil, she says. Hold for up to 5 minutes.

Douse that fever. Wet a washcloth in cool water and wipe down your face and neck, says Don Beckstead, M.D., a family-practice physician in Altoona, Pennsylvania. As the water evaporates, it takes some of the heat from your skin. If it makes you feel better, you can leave the cloth on your forehead until it warms up. Reapply a freshly cooled cloth as many times as you like. But if your temperature reaches 101°F, acetaminophen is generally the drug of choice, advises Dr. Beckstead.

Massage away the mucus. To help clear mucus from your chest, put one or two drops of eucalyptus oil, available in health food stores, on your thumbs and massage the upper portion of the soles of your feet, says Muryn. (If you have sensitive skin, mix the oil with your favorite body cream.) Hold your foot in the palm of one hand while using the other to knead the flat area just below the toes. "Always massage up, toward the toes," Muryn says.

Apply warm heat. If you don't have a fever, take a nice, warm soak in the tub to help ease the tired, achy muscles that are especially prevalent with the flu, says Dr. Beckstead. Twenty to 30 minutes is all it takes to start feeling better. Plus, the steam might help open up a clogged nose.

Use the snooze treatment. Try to sleep at least 8 hours during the night, and get as much rest as possible during the day, even if you don't actually sleep, says Dr. Beckstead. There's no better way to relax your body and recoup some of the energy that will help you fight viral invaders.

If you have trouble getting to sleep because you're really congested, raise your head with a few extra pillows to help you breathe more easily. Lying on your back with your head elevated, you might prevent mucus from draining down your throat and disrupting your breathing. As for when you should sleep, "Your body will let you know when it's tired," says Dr. Beckstead. Your job is to listen.

Take it slow when you start again. If you've had flu or the below-the-neck symptoms of a bad cold (like a hacking cough), you can resume exercising when those symptoms subside, advises Dr. Primos. But ease back into it, or you could end up sick again. For every day that you were sick, exercise at a lower intensity for 2 days upon your return. If you were sick for 3 days, for instance, take it easy for the first 6 days that you work out after your illness.

Commuter's Back

First the bad news: Since 1987, traffic on American roads has increased by 40 percent. Now the worse news: The number of miles of new roads has increased by only 1 percent. Translation: All of us—especially folks who commute by car—are going to spend more time trapped behind the wheel and thus be more at risk for the aches and pains that are an occupational hazard of driving.

But fear not. There's good news as well. You can avoid the pothole of back pain by turning your chariot into a workout gym on wheels.

Mapping Out a Back Strategy

Here are some stress busters and posture promoters to help you steer clear of back attacks.

Strike the right pose. Proper posture is the key to guaranteeing the long ride doesn't charge tolls on your back, says Jane Sullivan-Durand, M.D., a behavioral medicine physician in Contoocook, New Hampshire.

"When you climb into a car, you lose the stabilizing

forces of the buttocks and legs to hold you up," says Dr. Sullivan-Durand. "You must count on your abdomen, back, and vertebrae. That's where good posture comes in." Here is her plan for perfect driving posture.

- Sit in an upright position.
- Make sure that the small of your back is flush with the back of the car seat. Use a small pillow or cushion if you need extra support.
- Use your stomach muscles to hold in your torso.

To help maintain your posture, Dr. Sullivan-Durand suggests that you adjust your rearview and side mirrors so that they are best viewed when you are sitting up straight.

Here are some more techniques for saving your back the next time you hit the road.

Stay in motion. No time to exercise? Simply plug in Karkicks. The 60-minute audiotape, created by Natalie Manor of Merrimack, New Hampshire, and endorsed by the New Hampshire Safety Council, lets you exercise your back and the rest of your body while traveling from here to there. The tape can be purchased by writing to Karkicks, P.O. Box 1508, Merrimack, NH 03054.

"One of the great things about Karkicks is that it is always reminding you to tuck in your tummy," says Dr. Sullivan-Durand. "When you do that, you take strain off your lower back."

Shrug off traffic. To relieve tension in the upper back, Dr. Sullivan-Durand suggests this shoulder shimmy from Karkicks.

- Keep both hands on the steering wheel.
- Lift both shoulders toward your ears as if you were shrugging, then roll them backward. Hold for a few seconds.
- Try 10 shoulder shrugs every hour during your commute.

Hit the ceiling. Give your total back a lift and increase bloodflow with this upside-down pushup offered by Karkicks, says Dr. Sullivan-Durand (don't forget to close the sunroof first).

- Keep your right hand on the steering wheel.
- Place your left hand, palm side up, flat on the car's ceiling (be sure that you can still see through the windshield and in the mirrors).
- Push your left hand into the ceiling.
- Hold the pressure for a few seconds, then relax. Do 10 of these pushups.
- Repeat these steps with your right hand while you hold the wheel with your left hand.

Stretch while you drive. Kimbra Kimball, a licensed massage therapist and co-owner of Massage Therapeutics in Allentown, Pennsylvania, suggests this exercise.

- Extend your left hand toward the windshield.
- Lean toward the steering wheel just until you feel a stretch in your back and shoulders. Don't touch the wheel with your chest.
- Hold this stretch for 30 seconds and repeat three or four times. Be sure to keep your head up and your eyes on the road while doing this stretch.
- Switch hands and repeat three or four times with your other arm. "You're elongating the back, stretching those very long muscles on both sides of the spine," explains Kimball.

Unclench that steering wheel. Have you ever felt aches in your fingers, wrists, and back after a two-hour plow through traffic? Maybe it's because you were unconsciously putting a death grip on the steering wheel.

"When we drive, we increase our muscle tension because we maintain this vigilant state of driving defen-

Trying Some Kicks on Route 66

They drove from southern California to eastern Pennsylvania without a drop of coffee. More important, Kimbra Kimball and a friend covered the 4,000-mile trek in 8 days—without a single back twinge, ache, or spasm.

Their secret? The pair kept their backs and bodies limber by doing exercises in the car, at rest stops, at gas stations, and along the shoulder of the road, says Kimball, a licensed massage therapist who relocated from Los Angeles to Allentown, Pennsylvania.

At roadside stops, they took turns lying on the front seat with their feet dangling out the open passenger door. Kimball did leg lifts, which stretch the quadriceps and the abdomen, then curl-ups, which help stretch the back muscles and relieve tension. She recommends doing two or three leg lifts and two or three curl-ups, holding each for 30 seconds.

"The key thing for anyone who spends a lot of time in the car is to get out and do stretches," says Kimball. "The stretching movements bring oxygen into the body and brain. They clear your head, making you feel energized and revived."

sively," explains Dr. Sullivan-Durand. To fight it, she suggests this exercise.

Place both hands on the steering wheel. Curl your hands over the top (but don't let go). Squeeze your hands for a few seconds, then relax them. Remember to breathe in through your nose and out through your mouth as you relax your muscles to deepen the relaxation. Repeat this movement 10 times every hour.

Shift into rear. An important rule: Never neglect your buttocks on a long car ride. Dr. Sullivan-Durand and

Rodger Koppa, Ph.D., transportation researcher at the Texas Transportation Institute and industrial engineering professor at Texas A&M University in College Station, say this exercise from Karkicks works well. The payoff is both a relaxed back and a firmer backside.

Lift your rear slightly from the seat by squeezing the buttock muscles. Hold for 10 seconds, then drop it. If you are truly talented, try lifting your right buttock slightly and then letting it drop. Do 10 lifts, alternating your right and left buttocks. Keep your stomach tucked in, and sit up straight.

Let the luggage wait. Don't be in a big hurry to leap out of your car and hoist that heavy suitcase out after a long trip, says Dr. Sullivan-Durand. "Your spinal column needs a little flexing before it can take the stress of lifting something heavy." She recommends doing a full-body stretch first, like an exaggerated yawn. In a standing position, raise your arms over your head, bend to one side, and hold for 10 seconds, then repeat on the other side.

Another good stretch for your neck, shoulders, and back is to stand with your knees bent and roll forward slowly. Start with your neck and progress with each vertebra of your spine until your waist is bent and your head is almost touching your knees. You can place your hands on your thighs for support if necessary.

Now you're ready to deal with that suitcase. First, move your suitcase to the edge of the trunk. Then, with your back straight, bend your knees and lift it out.

Diverticulitis

It's a series of intestinal developments just waiting for trouble to happen.

Maybe you've been straining a lot during bowel movements, or maybe the walls of your colon have weakened a bit. Little pouches and sacs called diverticula have formed in the lining of your colon.

In these little dead-end streets, debris may become trapped. When those troublemakers aren't flushed out of your system, they ferment, decay, and inflame tissues—and you have diverticulitis.

People who develop diverticulitis often have had previous symptoms of constipation and difficult bowel movements with hard stools, according to Kristin Stiles, N.D., a naturopathic doctor at the Complementary Medicine and Healing Arts Center in Vestal, New York.

The problem announces itself with a wide range of symptoms. Even your doctor may be puzzled about the exact cause. Among the signs are alternating diarrhea and constipation, gas, bloating, and chronic cramping and pain in the intestines. Since these mimic many of the symptoms of irritable bowel syndrome (IBS), it takes some medical sleuthing to determine what you have. After treatment to help reduce the inflammation, your doctor will probably want to do a follow-up colon examination to find out whether diverticulitis is really the problem.

Healing Your Irritation

Once you know that you have diverticulitis, your doctor may help you find ways to improve your diet. Some supplements can help you recover more quickly. Here's what experts suggest.

Soothe inflamed membranes. When you're in the throes of diverticulitis, your immediate problems are inflammation, infection, and irritation of the colon. Several herbs, called demulcents, have the ability to soothe and coat mucous membranes, says Pamela Taylor, N.D., a naturopathic doctor in Moline, Illinois.

Some health food stores carry a naturopathic herbal combination known as Robert's Formula that is very good for gastrointestinal irritation, she says. The combination includes herbs such as slippery elm, marshmallow root, and geranium. It may also contain echinacea and goldenseal, two botanical ingredients that help boost your immune system.

Robert's Formula is produced by a number of different companies, with varying combinations of ingredients. It is generally available in capsules or as a tincture. Simply follow the directions on the label, recommends Dr. Taylor. A usual dose is either two "00" capsules three times a day or 10 to 15 drops of tincture 20 minutes before each meal and at bedtime, she says.

You can also take some of the herbs separately. Slippery elm alone is a powerful demulcent. Usually you'll find it in 100-milligram capsules. Take three a day, recommends

Melissa Metcalfe, N.D., a naturopathic doctor in Los Angeles.

Turmeric also works well as an anti-inflammatory, she says; try taking a 200- to 400-milligram capsule twice a day.

Chamomile is another good anti-inflammatory that's soothing to gastrointestinal tissues. Dr. Metcalfe suggests taking two 400- to 500-milligram capsules three times a day.

You can continue to take any of these supplements as long as you have problems with diverticulitis, she says.

Kill the infection. Infection is always a concern with diverticulitis. If it is not controlled, doctors sometimes recommend surgery to remove affected portions of the intestine. You can help your body fight any infection in the colon by taking a combination of echinacea and goldenseal, says Dr. Stiles.

Both herbs have anti-inflammatory and antibacterial properties. "You don't want to take either of these herbs for too long, however. I'd recommend 2 weeks on and 2 weeks off until the infection subsides," says Dr. Stiles. "You can quickly build up a tolerance to echinacea, so it becomes less effective."

A typical dose is one 200- to 250-milligram capsule of echinacea and one 50- to 60-milligram capsule of goldenseal three or four times a day, she suggests. Health food stores and some drugstores also carry combination capsules. Alternatively, you can take 10 to 15 drops of an extract of each herb in water or juice three or four times a day, with or without food.

Heal damaged membranes with vitamins. Dr. Taylor sometimes recommends that her patients take vitamins A, E, and C and a chelated form of zinc. Many companies market these nutrients in a single supplement, says Dr. Taylor. She uses the following daily amounts, based on a

A Soothing Spice

If you like Indian food, you're in luck. Turmeric, the main ingredient in curry powder, is a powerful anti-inflammatory that can help reduce the puffiness and soreness of irritated tissue. Plus, it's a digestive aid. Naturopathic doctors sometimes recommend it as a treatment for diverticulitis.

Indian doctors use it for many inflammatory conditions, from rheumatoid arthritis to sprains. They sometimes make poultices of turmeric that are applied directly to sore muscles and painful joints. In animal studies, it has been shown to reduce the amount of gas that's produced in the intestine and increase the secretion of gastric juices. It protects the stomach, possibly helping to prevent ulcers.

Although turmeric has several active ingredients, curcumin seems to be the most important for medicinal purposes. In fact, because it comes in a highly concentrated form, curcumin alone—available in capsules at health food stores—can be more effective than turmeric.

body weight of 150 pounds: 5,000 to 10,000 international units (IU) of vitamin A in the form of fish oil, 200 to 500 milligrams of vitamin C, 100 to 400 IU of vitamin E, and 15 to 30 milligrams of chelated zinc. You'll need to check with a naturopathic doctor to determine the dosages appropriate for your weight and follow his advice on when to take the supplement.

Prevent it with fiber. "When I see this problem, it's usually because the person is eating a high-fat, high-sugar, low-fiber diet," says Dr. Stiles. "I immediately get him onto a high-fiber diet."

You should consume between 25 and 30 grams of soluble and insoluble fiber each day, advises Dr. Stiles, and she advocates getting most of that through diet. Fiber is found in fruits and vegetables, legumes, and grains, like whole wheat, oats, and rye. "I wouldn't recommend that you eat foods with any seeds, like sesame or sunflower. You don't want a lot of hard stuff in the stool passing through this really irritated area," says Dr. Metcalfe. When your colon is very irritated, she adds, it may be best to start out with a fiber supplement rather than eat a lot of rough fiber, like bran.

If you're not getting the recommended amount of fiber from food, Dr. Stiles recommends taking 2 tablespoons daily of a fiber supplement that contains psyllium.

Since fiber absorbs large amounts of water, make sure that you drink plenty, whether you're increasing your food fiber or taking supplemental fiber. Dr. Stiles suggests that you drink 8 to 10 8-ounce glasses of water daily. The water adds bulk to the stool and helps soften it for easier transit through the colon.

As you recover from diverticulitis, the inflammation will heal, but you still need to pay attention to the factors that may have contributed to the problem in the first place. Be sure to maintain a low-fat, high-fiber diet, exercise regularly, and drink adequate amounts of water, says Dr. Stiles.

Elbow Pain

A riddle: What does your elbow have in common with a Thoroughbred horse farm?

Answer: They're both pretty stable joints.

But seriously, folks . . . in general, the elbow—the muscles and tendons that connect three bones, the radius, the ulna, and the humerus—is a fairly sturdy structure. But when things do go awry in there, you suddenly become painfully aware of how often you bend and bang your arm. Elbow ache is a nuisance.

Two of the most common elbow afflictions are quite sporty: tennis elbow and its less famous but sometimes equally obnoxious sibling, golfer's elbow.

Elbow pain can make turning a doorknob or wringing out a towel difficult, says Dr. Anderson. Here's how to get immediate relief.

Apply a hot ointment. Made from a derivative of hot peppers (capsaicin) and commonly used for shingles, Zostrix is extremely effective at zapping elbow pain, says Craig Hersh, M.D., a sports injuries specialist at the Sports Medicine Center in Fort Lee, New Jersey. This over-the-counter topical ointment, available at most drugstores, works as a temporary anesthetic when rubbed on the sore area, he says. "It doesn't work on inflammation—it works at the nerve level, blocking the transmission of pain."

Cool down that elbow. You can soothe that sore elbow by rubbing it with a paper cup filled with ice (fill the cup with water and freeze it) or a resealable plastic bag filled with ice cubes and wrapped in a towel. "Just don't leave the ice on any longer than 10 to 20 minutes," says Susan Perry, a physical therapist specializing in sports medicine at the Fort Lauderdale Sports Medicine Clinic in Fort Lauderdale, Florida. Apply the ice no more than four times a day, with at least an hour between icings, she suggests. A bag of frozen peas (or other small vegetables) also works as a reusable elbow ice pack, she says.

Tennis Elbow, Anyone?

You don't have to be a Wimbledon qualifier to get tennis elbow. Anyone who repeatedly rotates the elbow or flexes the wrist while gripping a heavy object is at risk. That includes people who work with tools, do a lot of gardening, or just tote a heavy briefcase. Tennis elbow is the inflammation of the wrist extensor muscles where they attach to the outer knob of the elbow's upper arm bone. It's the most common form of chronic elbow pain.

"Tennis elbow is a catch-all term for pain in the outer elbow joint," says Dale Anderson, M.D., an urgent-care physician in Minneapolis and author of health humor books such as *The Orchestra Conductor's Secret to Health and Long Life.*

One Swedish study showed that exercises that stretch the forearm muscles improved range of motion and reduced elbow pain. These exercises may help you ace tennis elbow.

Stretch those muscles. Here's a stretch that's a good warmup for elbow activity, according to Michael Ciccotti, M.D., an orthopedic surgeon and director of sports medicine at the Rothman Institute at Thomas Jefferson University in Philadelphia.

- Stretch your left arm in front of you, keeping your elbow straight and your palm down.
- Slowly bend your wrist downward until your fingers point toward the floor.
- Place your right hand on top of your left hand and gently press until you feel a tension stretch in your left forearm. Hold for 15 seconds.
- Repeat the same steps with your right arm.

Give your elbow a flex. Jeffrey Willson, a certified athletic trainer at K Valley Orthopedics in Kalamazoo, Michigan, suggests this basic stretch. He recommends doing this exercise four or five times a day, holding the stretch for 10 seconds at a time.

- Begin with your aching arm hanging at your side.
- Bend your elbow to 90 degrees so that your palm is facing up.
- Slowly rotate your palm to face the ground.
- Flex your wrist by bending your fingers toward the underside of your forearm.
- Finally, keeping your wrist flexed, straighten your elbow.

Try the tendon glide. This exercise will help alleviate and possibly prevent elbow pain, according to Robert Markison, M.D., a hand surgeon and associate clinical professor of surgery at the University of California, San Francisco. "It's a good stretching exercise for all the tendons in the wrist and elbows," he says, "especially before you plan to do a lot of computer keyboard work."

- Extend one arm, palm up, in front of you.
- Use your other hand to pull back on the fingers of the extended hand, bending your hand at the wrist.
- Let go of your fingers and turn the extended arm over so that the palm faces down.
- Again pull back on your fingers with the opposite hand, bending at the wrist.
- Repeat with the other arm, then do the entire sequence once more.

Master massage. To relax the muscles surrounding your elbow, massage your forearm, suggests Meir Schneider, Ph.D., a licensed massage therapist, founder of the Center and School for Self-Healing in San Francisco, and creator of the Meir Schneider Self-Healing Method.

Starting at your wrist, make large, unhurried circles with your fingertips, kneading the muscles up to your elbow. Massage both the front and the back of your forearm. Alternatively, you can grasp your forearm with your thumb on the underside of your wrist and your fingers on top and massage both surfaces at the same time. Knead in circles with your thumb and fingertips. The total massage should take about 5 minutes to complete.

Golfer's Elbow

Golfer's elbow is the flip side of tennis elbow. While tennis elbow is a problem with the muscles that help the wrist straighten and extend, golfer's elbow affects the flexor muscles, which help the wrist and elbow bend. This problem isn't limited to Tiger Woods wannabes, according to Dr. Anderson. The golf moniker stems from the fact that golfers who dig up too much of the grass with their swings often strain their flexors.

Try the swan position. To assuage the pain, try this "fold and hold" exercise recommended by Dr. Anderson. If you position your wrist and forearm correctly, he says, the tender spot should improve by at least 75 percent.

- Fold your upper arm close to your body by bending your elbow into a tight angle. Bring the back of your wrist close to your shoulder.
- Bend and flex your wrist with the fingertips pointing downward. The palm of your hand should face the ground. Your arm should resemble a swan, with your hand as the head.
- Use your other hand to fine-tune your wrist and forearm into the most pain-free position.
- Place your other hand on top of the hand that's bent.
- Hold for 90 seconds, then release slowly.

Making Your Elbows Stronger

Here are two more ideas for beefing up your elbows.

Get a grip. To work the elbow muscles, grab a hand gripper or squeeze a tennis ball, says Dr. Ciccotti. Grip and hold for 5 seconds, then release. Repeat this 15 times. The steady motion of gripping, squeezing, and releasing works the flexor and extensor muscles in the hand and elbow. If you feel sharp pain in your elbow or wrist, however, stop the exercise, he says.

Resist yourself. Hold your left arm in front of you with the palm facing down. Make a fist and bend your left wrist upward. Cup your right hand over your left fist and try to push straight down with your right hand as you resist the downward force with your left fist. Tense the muscles for 10 seconds, then relax. Try five times, then switch hands and repeat.

Doing this exercise two or three times a day can bolster the muscles around your elbows and wrists, says Dr. Ciccotti.

Fibromyalgia

The Platters spun to the top of the charts in 1955 with "The Great Pretender." Today it could be the theme song for fibromyalgia, an often misdiagnosed condition whose symptoms mimic those associated with arthritis, multiple sclerosis, chronic fatigue syndrome, and even tennis elbow.

Fibromyalgia is an irritation of the connective tissue that supports structures throughout the body. Although its symptoms are clear—debilitating muscle aches, stiffness, and fatigue sometimes accompanied by headaches and a case of the blues—its causes aren't. If your shoulder aches for no apparent reason, for instance, you might have fibromyalgia. "It spans the spectrum of pain from annoying to disabling," says James Stark, M.D., a physiatrist at the Center for Sports Medicine in San Francisco.

Studies suggest that people are born with an inherited tendency toward fibromyalgia, and it may be brought on by physical or emotional trauma, stress, or exposure to environmental toxins, including tobacco smoke. This condition, like all chronic pain, may also cause depression.

Attack It from the Inside Out

"Fibromyalgia tends to manifest itself like chronic fatigue syndrome, but the pain is the predominant factor. Also, people who have fibromyalgia tend to be malnourished," says Hope Fay, N.D., a naturopathic doctor in Seattle. "There are lots of different theories, treatments, and supplements out there. Some work for some people; others don't. It is one of those conditions that you try to treat very broadly."

You may get relief with these supplements.

Support your immune system. Recovering from fibromyalgia can be a lengthy process, says Elizabeth Wotton, N.D., a naturopathic doctor at Compass Family Health Center in Plymouth, Massachusetts. She likes to prescribe the herb astragalus, a long-term immune booster. Dr. Wotton recommends taking 1 teaspoon of astragalus liquid extract three times a day. You can also take astragalus capsules. If the supplements are 500 milligrams, a typical dose would be one or two capsules three times a day with meals.

"Astragalus begins to build up the immune system to provide support on a long-term basis. It's really good for this type of chronic condition because it gives you some stability," she says. "You should take it for at least 4 to 6 months."

Get a lift with ginseng. Deep weariness is one of fibromyalgia's most nagging symptoms. To give her patients a lift, Dr. Wotton recommends ginseng. "It's a tonic herb that makes you feel less run-down," she says.

She recommends 1 to 2 teaspoons of the liquid extract twice a day or one 200-milligram capsule twice a day. But don't take ginseng after 2:00 P.M., she cautions, because it can keep you awake at night. It may also cause irritability if taken with caffeine or other stimulants.

Take Magnesium for Your Muscles

Many fibromyalgia patients seem to have low levels of magnesium, which may be a significant cause of their muscle pain, says Dr. Wotton. By adding magnesium to your diet, you could help relieve that sore, tired feeling. Look in health food stores for a magnesium supplement that contains malic acid, she says. Take 200 milligrams three times a day for 4 to 6 months.

Get the right kind of fat. Reducing any kind of inflammation usually brings about some improvement, says Dr. Fay. In fibromyalgia, there is clearly inflammation in the muscles and probably in the intestinal tract as well. You may be able to lessen inflammation throughout your body by reducing your consumption of meat and taking essential fatty acid supplements that do not contribute to inflammation, Dr. Fay says.

She suggests a 1,000-milligram capsule of evening primrose oil three or four times a day. Some people do better if they start with small amounts and increase with time, says Dr. Fay. You can take this preparation at this dosage for 3 to 6 months and then gradually begin to cut back, she advises.

Increase your vitamins and minerals. Malnourishment seems to be part of the problem for many fibromyalgia patients. Either their diets are quite poor, food allergies are involved, or the people just aren't extracting enough energy and nutrients from food, says Dr. Fay.

She tells her patients to cut out coffee, sugar, and refined foods and start on healthier diets that include more fresh fruits and vegetables, more whole grains, and less red meat.

Also, she suggests that they take multivitamin/mineral supplements that provide nutrients in amounts higher than the Daily Values.

Muscle Stretches

One thing doctors are sure about is that regular exercise routines emphasizing muscle stretches, low-impact aerobics, and relaxation can control the pain of fibromyalgia. Here are some exercises tailored to those three areas.

Stand in the doorway. The doorway stretch prepares your muscles for exertion, says Devin Starlanyl, M.D., a West Chesterfield, New Hampshire, physician and author who has fibromyalgia.

- Stand in the middle of a doorway, facing forward, with your arms outstretched and your hands resting firmly on each side of the doorjamb at shoulder height.
- Take a step forward, and feel the stretch across your chest. Hold the stretch for 30 to 60 seconds.
- Return to the starting position, and move your hands farther down on the doorjamb. Again, take a step forward and stretch.

This is a good stretching exercise to do once or twice a day, Dr. Starlanyl says.

Massage those aches. Researchers at the University of Miami recommend massages for people with fibromyalgia. In one study, 10 people with fibromyalgia received 30-minute massages twice a week for 5 weeks. They experienced decreased anxiety and less stress, pain, stiffness, and fatigue.

Play wall ball. You don't need a racquet or a net to do this tennis ball exercise, recommended by Dr. Starlanyl.

First of all, identify the tender spots, or "trigger points," where the pain seems to originate. Place a tennis or

Do You Have Pain at the Tender Points?

Since fibromyalgia is so difficult to identify, the Arthritis Foundation offers these helpful clues.

- Fibromyalgia is a syndrome characterized by generalized muscle pain and fatigue. It does not affect the joints.
- Pain may start in one part of the body and seem to gradually spread all over.
- People describe fibromyalgia pain as burning, radiating, gnawing, sore, stiff, and achy.
- People with fibromyalgia experience soreness and tenderness in at least 11 of 18 identified tender points on the body, including the elbows, knees, waist, and points around the neck.
- Nine out of 10 people with fibromyalgia experience fatigue caused by interrupted sleep.
- No single lab test or x-ray can diagnose fibromyalgia.
- The cause is unknown, but doctors say that stress, physical injury, smoking, poor posture, and other factors may play a role.

lacrosse ball on that trigger point, and apply pressure by leaning against a wall or lying on the floor with the ball between your body and the firm surface. When you compress the trigger point, liquids in that area are forced out. When the pressure is lifted, the blood and other body fluids rush back in and flush the area, bringing needed oxygen and nutrients to the tissues.

If the trigger point is under one buttock, for instance, here's how to apply pressure with a tennis ball.

- Lie on your back with your knees bent and your feet flat on the floor. Your knees should not touch.
- Raise your hips slightly and slide a tennis ball under one of them.
- Move your hip down and rest on the ball for 30 to 60 seconds. You can expect to feel some pain, but you can control the pressure that you exert. If you roll the ball around, the pain should ease.

Easy-Does-It Aerobics

Regular low-impact aerobic exercise for at least 20 minutes a day increases bloodflow to the muscles and boosts endorphins, the body's natural pain fighters, says Dr. Stark. Here are some low-sweat, non-joint-jarring exercises to combat pain from fibromyalgia.

Try a spin. Stationary cycling can reduce tenderness and promote sound sleep, says Dr. Stark. He urges people who have been inactive to gradually ease into cycling or a similar type of program after conferring with their doctors.

Rock away the pain. Never underestimate the aerobic benefits of your favorite living room rocker, says Dr. Stark. Maybe you can gently rock back and forth through your favorite half-hour sitcom. The rocking action activates leg muscles and lessens the effects of immobility, he says.

Stride often. A 20-minute walk, properly executed, can do wonders for fibromyalgia, says Dr. Starlanyl. She offers these walking tips.

- Keep your head held over your shoulders for balance.
- Shift your weight from your heels to the balls of your feet to your toes as you step forward.
- Push off each step from your toes, using your calf muscles.

- Move briskly, but be able to maintain a conversation without being short of breath.

Reach Relaxation

These exercises may help both physically and emotionally.

Guide pain away. Visualize the muscle pain in physical terms such as "a burning fire" or "a terrible monster gnawing on your bones." By mentally extinguishing the flames or taming the monster, you may be able to reduce pain, says Norman Harden, M.D., a neurologist and director of the Center for Pain Studies at the Rehabilitation Institute of Chicago.

Hug your dog or cat. A friendly head scratch or hug can make a dog drool in delight and a cat purr with pride. Pets help reduce pain, tension, and stress, says Dr. Harden.

Take up tai chi. This ancient Chinese martial art enhances mind-body connection, balance, and harmony, says Dr. Stark. Its slow, fluid, circular motions in graceful sequences strengthen muscles and improve coordination and balance. Think of it as a moving meditation, he adds.

Foot Pain

If you've got achy feet, you'll never squawk alone. Three out of every four Americans share your problem in their pedal extremities. It's no wonder. Our feet are intricate systems, featuring 26 bones and 33 joints each, and the average person takes 8,000 to 10,000 steps a day. That's a lot of stress on our poor little doggies.

Foot pain is also an unfair affliction, in that it affects a lot more women than men. According to the American Podiatric Medical Association, women have about four times as many foot problems. Wearing high heels is often the culprit.

Some foot pain is simple to diagnose, particularly if it's caused by ill-fitting shoes. Arthritis and circulation problems may also be culprits. If bloodflow is compromised in any way, our feet, at the far reaches of the circulatory system, feel it most acutely.

Nip Pain in the Bud

Regardless of why your feet hurt, here are some soothing strategies.

Stomp on pain. Nonsteroidal anti-inflammatory drugs (NSAIDs) such as ibuprofen (Advil) can relieve the pain and swelling of most types of foot pain. Follow package directions. This is a temporary fix, however. You don't want to stay on over-the-counter painkillers for more than a few weeks, advises Tzvi Bar-David, D.P.M., podiatrist with Columbia-Presbyterian Medical Center in New York City. So make sure to try other strategies to relieve your specific foot problem.

Make ginger a habit. Fresh ginger is a great remedy for arthritis and other pain related to swelling because it's a natural anti-inflammatory, says Neal Barnard, M.D., author of *Foods That Fight Pain* and president of the Physicians Committee for Responsible Medicine in Washington, D.C. Though you don't have to use a lot of it to get significant relief, you do have to take it regularly, he says.

Buy fresh ginger at the supermarket. Mince up ½ to 1 teaspoon per day. Either put it in your food as a flavoring or mix it into some water and swallow it like a pill. Cloves, garlic, and turmeric, though less studied, have shown similar effects in some people, according to Dr. Barnard.

Rub hot peppers on them. Over-the-counter creams made from capsaicin, the active ingredient in hot peppers, can relieve arthritis and other foot pain, says Dr. Barnard. The lotion may at first cause a burning sensation, which decreases the more you use the stuff. Rub just enough to lightly cover the affected area on your feet whenever you feel pain. Wash your hands thoroughly after each application, and keep the cream away from your eyes and other mucous membranes. It can really burn.

Soak them. Treat your feet to a soak in Epsom salts and warm water. The soak can drain swollen tissues and help relieve pressure. Follow the directions on the package, which is usually 1 tablespoon of Epsom salts dissolved in each quart of water.

Put your feet in motion. For many foot faults, especially arthritis and circulation aches, motion is a great pain-fighting weapon. To take arms against throbbing feet, experts suggest three steps.

1. Do low-impact exercise regularly—about 30 minutes three or four times a week. Try bicycling or swimming.
2. Do stretching exercises.
3. Do strengthening exercises.

Healing with Heel Stretches

Heel pain is a common complaint among foot patients. Frequently, the source of the pain is a condition called plantar fasciitis, named after the plantar fascia, a flat ligament band on the underside of the foot. The plantar fascia, which acts like a bowstring to maintain the arch of the foot, can become inflamed when it's repeatedly placed under tension. The irritation can be caused by being overweight, by standing for long periods, or by excessive running or walking.

The pain may progress from a dull, intermittent heel ache to a sharp, persistent pain. Classically, it's worse in the morning with the first few steps you take, says Steven Lawrence, M.D., an orthopedic surgeon at the Lancaster Orthopedic Group in Pennsylvania.

Simple stretching exercises relieve heel pain in many cases. "The key to treating plantar fasciitis is stretching," says Thomas Meade, M.D., an orthopedic surgeon and medical director of the Allentown Sports Medicine Clinic and Human Performance Center in Pennsylvania. He suggests these heel-health exercises.

When to See a Doctor

If foot pain persists for more than 2 to 3 days, seek professional care to rule out any serious problems such as infection or circulatory problems, advises Leonard A. Levy, D.P.M., professor of podiatric medicine and past president of the California College of Podiatric Medicine in San Francisco. People who may be at special risk—the elderly, people with diabetes, and those with circulatory problems, for instance—should seek medical attention if the pain persists for more than several hours.

Take the first step. Here is a do-anywhere stretch to combat heel pain. You should feel a stretch in the calf and plantar fascia, but Dr. Meade warns that you shouldn't do this stretch if you feel pain. If you stand on a stepstool (or nail together some two-by-fours to make a portable step), you can do this exercise while brushing your teeth, washing dishes, or standing and watching television, Dr. Meade notes.

- Stand with your legs straight on the bottom step of a flight of stairs, holding on to the railing. Or use your portable step and a table for support.
- Stand so that the ball of the afflicted foot is on the edge of the step. Put the other foot flat on the step.
- Slowly drop your heel until you feel a stretch in the back of your calf muscle.
- Hold the stretch for at least 20 seconds. Repeat 8 to 12 times and then switch to the other foot.

Use a therapeutic towel. This exercise is designed to stretch inflamed plantar fascia tissue and relieve pressure on the nerves in the foot, says Dr. Meade. It can help relieve pain and in general tune up your feet to keep future discomfort away. "Let pain be your guide," he adds. "This should feel tight but not painful."

- Lie on your back with your legs straight.
- Loop a towel around the ball of your sore foot and gently but firmly pull the towel toward you. You'll feel tension in the bottom of your foot.
- Hold the stretch for 20 seconds. Repeat 10 times and then do the same with your other foot.

If the Shoe Doesn't Fit

The right-fitting slipper brought Cinderella and the prince together. A properly fitted shoe also reduces the risk of bunions, corns, calluses, hammertoes, and other foot maladies, according to the American Orthopaedic Foot and Ankle Society (AOFAS).

Here are some shoe-buying tips from the AOFAS that will help you have pain-free feet.

- Judge the shoe by the way it fits your foot and not by the size marked inside the shoe. One brand's size 6 is another brand's size 7.
- Have your feet measured regularly, because foot sizes change as you grow older.
- Shop for shoes at the end of the day, when your feet are largest.
- Make sure the ball of your foot fits comfortably into the widest part of the shoe.
- Stand during the fitting process. Check that there is ⅜ to ½ inch of space for your longest toe at the end of each shoe.
- Don't buy tight shoes and expect them to stretch to fit later.

Do the golf ball massage. It's too rainy to play 18 holes? Or maybe your foot hurts too much. Try this sporting stretch, suggested by Dr. Lawrence. It's great for people with plantar fasciitis, arch strain, and foot cramps. Simply place your foot on top of a golf ball on a flat surface, then roll the ball forward and backward across the underside of your foot for about 2 minutes. The ball provides a soothing, relaxing massage.

Rubbing the Right Way

A 5-minute foot massage can sometimes relieve discomfort as well as make you feel relaxed and rejuvenated, says Leonard A. Levy, D.P.M., professor of podiatric medicine and past president of the California College of Podiatric Medicine in San Francisco. Dr. Levy recommends following these steps.

- Sit comfortably in a chair or on the floor.
- Bring your right foot toward you, resting your right ankle on your left knee.
- Starting at the heel, press and knead the bottom of the foot with your fingers. Move up the middle of your foot, then veer over to your big toe and work across your foot to the little toe.
- Massage the pad under each toe.
- Gently squeeze each toe with your thumb and forefinger, moving each toe from side to side and gently stretching each toe out.
- Wrap your hands around your foot at the arch so that your thumbs are on your instep and your fingers on the other side of your foot. Knead your instep with your thumbs.
- Place the outer edge of your palm under the tips of your toes and gently pull back. As you flex your foot, hold for a few seconds, then let go and relax.

- Gently press the Achilles tendon (on the back of your heel) between your thumb and forefinger. Run your fingers up the back of your heel, ending above the ankle.
- Switch and repeat with your left foot.

Strengthening from Heel to Toe

You probably never think about the importance of strong feet. But no matter how much you use your tootsies, it always helps to keep them toned. Experts say that these exercises will banish pain and keep it away.

Take the towel challenge. Does your spouse simply drop the bath towel on the floor after showering? Turn this irritating habit into an exercise opportunity, suggests Dr. Meade. The goal here is to try to pick up the towel with your feet or, more precisely, with your toes.

Start at the near end of the towel and curl it toward you, using only your toes to scrunch it forward. Then try to pick the towel up with your toes and deposit it in the hamper or laundry basket.

For foot-fortifying variety, see if you can pick up 20 marbles or pencils, one at a time, with your toes and deposit them into a bowl. This motion strengthens the small muscles in the foot, which helps fight toe cramps, says Dr. Meade.

Try some toe tugs. For relief from toe cramps, doctors suggest looping a thick rubber band around all of the toes on one foot. Spread your toes apart, feeling the resistance from the rubber band. Try to hold this position for 5 to 10 seconds. Repeat 10 times before you switch and attempt the toe stretch with the opposite foot.

For variety, try a "toe-of-war" by placing the rubber band around both of your big toes and pulling them away from each other. Be sure to keep your heels in place. Hold for 5 to 10 seconds, and repeat 10 times.

Get on your tippies. Even if you can't do a pirouette like Mikhail Baryshnikov, this balletlike exercise will help fight toe cramps, says Dr. Levy.

You can stand or sit for this exercise, but put only as much weight on your toes as you can comfortably handle. First, remove your shoes, then do the following steps, one foot at a time. In a one-two-three sequence, rise to the ball of your foot, rise farther and point your toes, then curl your toes under. Try to hold each position for 5 to 10 seconds; repeat 10 times.

Gout

There was a time when people were reassured by the swelling and red-hot pain of a gouty foot. Since the pain zeroed in on a distant extremity—the big toe—it seemed to signify that all the nerves in the far reaches of the body were working well. Therefore, people surmised, maybe all was perfectly well with everything in between.

Gout is no all-clear signal, however. "That pain in the joint is the end result of a long breakdown process," says Luc Maes, D.C., N.D., a chiropractor and naturopathic doctor in Santa Barbara, California. It means that the kidneys are not doing a good job.

Your blood transports the chief troublemaker, uric acid. Like a traveler toting a heavy suitcase through an airport, blood that has a burden of excess uric acid begins looking for a dump site, says Dr. Maes. Down around the big toe, circulation is sluggish, and it's easy for the blood to drop its load. The uric acid deposited in the joint forms needle-shaped crystals that can trigger an inflammation so severe that even the weight of a bedsheet causes pain.

Purine-rich foods just make matters worse. Purines are chemicals found in foods such as alcohol, seafood, and organ meats. Normally they don't do any damage, but if you're prone to gout, these foods can cause crystal formation.

It helps to drink as much water as possible to help flush purines and uric acid from your system—and by all means eliminate purine-rich foods from your diet. It also helps to limit your intake of animal fats and refined carbohydrates, which increase the production of uric acid.

Along with those measures, nutritional and herbal supplements are good allies, say alternative medicine experts. Many can help improve the kidney, the liver, and the blood, according to Dr. Maes. Others can help fight inflammation. But he emphasizes that supplements can't make amends for a diet that includes lots of animal fats and refined carbohydrates. "If you eat a poor diet for a long time, your body gets too much of certain nutrients and not enough of others," he says.

Fight the flame with EPA. When you eat saturated fats—the kind in meat and dairy foods—you're inviting the overproduction of inflammatory chemicals. "Gout is a state of inflammation," says Dr. Maes. "Things are on fire."

Studies have shown that you can help reverse this pattern and correct the nutritional imbalance by taking fish oil or flaxseed oil. Fish-oil supplements are particularly rich in an omega-3 fatty acid called eicosapentaenoic acid (EPA), which discourages inflammation, says Priscilla Evans, N.D., a naturopathic doctor at the Community Wholistic Health Center in Chapel Hill, North Carolina. EPA is also available in flaxseed oil.

Like throwing a track switch to reroute a train, EPA reroutes the chemicals in your body early in the inflammation process. With the flick of that switch, the chemicals start to fight inflammation.

Supplements can't do the whole job, Dr. Evans emphasizes. "It's very important to cut back on saturated fats and on vegetable oils that promote inflammation. Just adding fish oil is not enough if you're still eating a lot of red meat and fat."

Dr. Maes advises people with gout to take 1,500 milligrams of fish oil a day, but not all at once. Divide the doses, and take the supplements with meals.

You should also take 400 to 1,200 international units of vitamin E a day with the fish oil, she says. It works along with the EPA to act as an anti-inflammatory and also serves as an antioxidant.

If you're a vegetarian or don't like fish, you may be able to get similar benefits by taking 1 to 2 tablespoons of flaxseed oil every day, says Dr. Maes. This oil contains alpha-linolenic acid, however, not the more valuable EPA, and the body converts only a portion of it to EPA.

Benefit from bromelain. Consider it an enzyme with an appetite. Bromelain, which comes from pineapple, is nature's anti-inflammatory medicine. Because it's an enzyme and enzymes help with digestion, you can take it with meals. You can also take it between meals. When you do, it works as an anti-inflammatory agent. "Bromelain inhibits those proteins that are promoting inflammation in the body. It kind of digests the products of inflammation," says Dr. Evans.

Dr. Evans recommends 500 milligrams of bromelain three times a day between meals to help reduce the inflammation during acute gout attacks. For milder cases of gout, you'll probably want to start out with a smaller dose since bromelain sometimes causes a burning feeling in the gut.

Although an attack of gout can last as long as a few weeks, you should take high doses of bromelain for only 4 to 5 days. After that, if the gout lingers, take 125 to 250 milligrams three times a day to control inflammation, advises Dr. Evans.

Put folic acid to work. Folic acid also has a dampening effect on uric acid production, studies show. This B vitamin gets in the way of the enzyme responsible for producing uric acid, and when that enzyme is blocked, uric acid production takes a nosedive. Folic acid won't resolve an acute attack, but in high doses it may help ward off future attacks.

For gout, the recommended dosage is 10,000 to 40,000 micrograms of folic acid daily. That's 25 to 100 times the Daily Value of 400 micrograms. Since that's far more than you should take without a prescription, you need to contact your physician if you would like to try folic acid as a preventive. Also, research has shown that you need to take some vitamin C along with the folic acid in order for it to work.

Get a boost from berries. Help in another form comes from bioflavonoid molecules, found in cherries, blueberries, and other fruits. In the 1950s, researchers discovered that cherries could decrease uric acid levels and prevent a gout attack. But you'd have to eat a lot of cherries—a ½-pound a day—to make a dent in gout.

For the same results, you can take a bioflavonoid supplement or 2,000 milligrams of berry extract a day, says Dr. Maes. The best are those that have a combination of all the bioflavonoids or the extracts of several different berries, he says.

Soothe with celery. When doctors prescribe a drug for gout relief, it's often allopurinal (Zyloprim), which controls uric acid levels. A natural alternative is celery seed extract, a supplement that acts as a diuretic, helping to flush fluids out of the system.

The pharmaceutical and the natural supplement were tested and compared by James A. Duke, Ph.D., botanical consultant, former ethnobotanist with the U.S. Department of Agriculture who specializes in medicinal plants, and author of *The Green Pharmacy*. After taking allopurinal, prescribed by his doctor for acute gout, Dr. Duke learned that celery seed extract might help just as much. He took two to four tablets of celery seed extract every day instead of allopurinol, and his attacks of gout disappeared.

Settle on nettle. Nettle, a natural antihistamine that has long been used by old-time herbalists to treat inflammation of the joints, also works as a diuretic to help to lower uric acid levels. "Nettle works as a blood cleanser and detoxifying agent," says Dr. Maes.

To get the full benefit, take 300 to 600 milligrams of a freeze-dried extract daily, he advises. Nettle may be used long-term, but Dr. Maes recommends using it for no more than 2 to 3 months at a time. Avoid tinctures of nettle, which contain alcohol and may aggravate gout.

Hangover

A wee bit too much wine at your cousin's wedding, and the next morning—o-o-o-ohhh—your punishment arrives: headache, nausea, thirst, muscle aches, and a big dose of despair.

The simple fact is, you've poisoned yourself. Alcohol causes your blood vessels to contract (headache), causes the buildup of poisons such as aldehydes and lactic acid in your cells (body aches), and dehydrates your entire system (thirst). All that hair-of-the-dog folk wisdom notwithstanding, there's only one real way to fix what you've done—get the alcohol out of your body as fast as possible.

Your body knows this. If you've really overindulged, vomiting may purge some of the stuff from your system. But by the morning after, even a good heave won't help with the alcohol that has already passed into your bloodstream. Exercise, however, may help speed recovery—if you're willing to breathe hard and sweat it out, says Melvin Williams, Ph.D., professor of exercise physiology at Old Dominion University in Norfolk, Virginia.

But there's one small problem. There's an anvil chorus

in your head. Lifting your head off the pillow barely seems possible. Still, the fact remains that if you pump up your circulation, respiration, and perspiration, the alcohol will leave your body more quickly and you'll feel better faster. Here, in ascending degree of difficulty, are a few easy exercises that can help exorcise the bourbon and get you back in the game.

Hydro-exercise. Not swimming in H_2O, but drinking it. Doctors agree that the most useful hangover antidote is w-a-t-e-r. "Alcohol makes you dehydrated, and the membranes of the brain scream for water," says Dan Hamner, M.D., a physiatrist and sports medicine specialist in New York City. Quaff some water before you go to sleep; Dr. Hamner recommends drinking at least 24 ounces of water before hitting the sheets.

Then, the next morning, have more. It not only helps with the rehydration of your body but may also help you

Running under the Influence

You may not feel like hard exercise if your head is about to explode, but sometimes a real physical challenge is just what you need to help with recovery.

Melvin Williams, Ph.D., professor of exercise physiology at Old Dominion University in Norfolk, Virginia, remembers one festive night in Russia. Drinks flowed and disco music pounded as his tour group celebrated their final night in Kiev.

"Normally, I just drink beer, but this was a special occasion," says Dr. Williams. "I didn't know how potent vodka can be."

He found out the next morning when a 7:00 A.M. wake-up call pried open his puffy, bloodshot eyes. Somehow, this marathoner willed himself out of bed, urinate. Anything that leaves your body takes at least a trace of the demon rum with it, says Dr. Hamner.

Respiro-exercises. Let your lungs help blow the alcohol out of your body, advises Dr. Williams. When you awaken—even before you brush your teeth—try taking deep breaths and blasting the alcohol-soaked air from your lungs. "You may get rid of the alcohol a little bit faster because you're ventilating more," he says.

Crawl to a sauna. More perspiration means a faster farewell for the toxins. "Alcohol is total poison for every cell in the body. A steam room should help for a hangover," Dr. Hamner says. Even a half-hour in a steamed-up bathroom might help a bit.

Beg for a massage. If you're lucky enough to have a loved one nearby, a gentle massage may help by getting your blood circulating, says Kimbra Kimball, a licensed massage therapist and co-owner of Massage Therapeutics

dressed, and ran his daily 8 miles before boarding the tour bus to the airport.

"I had a pounding headache for the first 5 or 6 minutes into the run, but by the end, I felt basically good," says Dr. Williams. He says that his heavy breathing while running possibly helped him excrete the poison in his bloodstream caused by heavy drinking.

Whether or not you're a runner, any kind of heart-pounding, blood-pumping exercise can help carry unwanted alcohol from your body, says Dan Hamner, M.D., a physiatrist and sports medicine specialist in New York City. "Try shadow boxing in front of a mirror for several minutes," he suggests. "That should get your heart rate up. You want to get that bad stuff out of you as fast as possible."

in Allentown, Pennsylvania. Make whatever deal you have to, but get your partner to minister to you softly. Here's the massage step-by-step.

Lie on your stomach with your arms at your sides. Your partner should:

1. Gently squeeze the underside of your heels, pushing the skin toward the end of the heel.
2. Move gradually up your legs with quick, gentle hand pumps that push your skin and muscles upward from the calves and thighs.
3. Keep heading north, massaging your buttocks, back, and shoulders.

Then flip over sunny-side up and have your partner give your stomach a gentle, circular massage in a clockwise direction. "By going clockwise, you are not resisting your normal body functions. And you are pushing everything in the right way for elimination," explains Kimball.

Stretch those muscles. When we drink too much, lactic acid and other poisons such as aldehydes build up in our muscles. Why? Because the liver gets overloaded trying to deal with all the toxins and can't keep up.

"Lactic acid is what makes you ache. Under a microscope, this molecule is abrasive to the body," explains Dr. Hamner. Try this soothing stretch to combat achiness from a hangover. You can do these movements even before you get out of bed in the morning.

- Lie flat on your back and stretch your hands and feet out. Reach for all four corners of the bed.
- Point your toes and stretch out your fingers.
- Slowly bring your left knee to your chest. Hold that pose for a few seconds and then slide your leg down.
- Repeat with your right leg.

Headache

Headaches come in many varieties. They can be big or little, frequent or infrequent, disabling or minor.

In sheer numbers, the tension headache rules with its dull, steady ache and muscle tenderness. In sheer power, the mighty migraine reigns with its arsenal of pulsating head throbs and the visual and speech disturbances and nausea that sometimes accompany it. But there are other kinds as well—the agonizing cluster headache, which pierces one temple with searing pain, or the rebound headache, which is literally the result of taking too much headache medicine. Headaches of various kinds can also be triggered by computer eyestrain, potent perfumes, and even ice cream.

Quick Pain Relief

According to the National Headache Foundation, about $4 billion a year goes toward over-the-counter pain relievers. Six out of every 10 people with headaches first reach for some nonprescription medication such as ibuprofen, according to a survey by Mediamark Research. But before you spend another buck on pills that put pain down, here are ways to heal headaches the drug-free way.

Apply ice to your head. Placing ice on your head while it hurts is one of the fastest and most effective ways to end a headache, according to Fred Sheftell, M.D., director of the New England Center for Headache in Stamford, Connecticut, and coauthor of *Headache Relief*. To put a deep freeze on your headache, he recommends getting an ice pack wrapped in a towel, or a bag of frozen vegetables or an ice pillow (available at drugstores). Place the ice on your forehead or on top of your head when you first notice any pain.

Try some heat on your neck. "Placing heat on the back of the head is great for relieving the pressure that accompanies tension headaches," says Glen Solomon, M.D., a headache specialist at the Cleveland Clinic Foundation in Cleveland and associate professor of medicine at Ohio State University in Columbus. He recommends a heating pad, a long, hot shower (turn the spray to the back of your neck), or a hot bath.

Pay attention to triggers. If you are prone to headaches, chances are you were born with a slightly different brain chemistry than people who don't get them. But that doesn't mean you're doomed, according to Dr. Sheftell. If you can avoid the pain triggers, you might be able to avoid the headaches.

Heading up Dr. Sheftell's Top Ten list of triggers are sensitivities to foods such as chocolate, certain food components such as alcohol and caffeine, and the food additive MSG. Other possible triggers are hormone fluctuations during the menstrual cycle, changes in the weather or season, sleeping late or not enough, bright lights, and odors. Last but certainly not least is that old bugbear stress.

Act Like a Turtle

This easy exercise—recommended by Roger Cady, M.D., director of the Headache Care Center in Springfield, Missouri—can help uncoil the tight muscles in your neck and shoulders and relieve a tension headache.

- While sitting or standing, inhale deeply.
- Tuck your chin in to your chest.
- Exhale fully and, as you do, raise your head and stick your chin out as far as you can. The curve of your neck should be exaggerated.

Do this chinning exercise three to five times, advises Dr. Cady. You may feel like a turtle, but you should also feel better.

Taming the Tension Headache

More than 90 percent of all headaches are tension headaches. The symptoms are inescapable: pain, usually on both sides of the head; a dull, steady ache; muscle soreness; and a run-down feeling. Here are some ways out of that nagging discomfort.

Find a rush-hour relaxer. For many people, the worst head racker crops up on the highway. "A lot of tension headaches are associated with neck tightness, sometimes triggered by scrunching up inside a car," says Joseph Primavera, Ph.D., a psychologist at the headache clinic at Thomas Jefferson University Hospital in Philadelphia.

To alleviate that tension, first loosen your grip on the steering wheel, suggests Dr. Primavera. Adjust your seat and posture so that you're sitting up as straight as possible. Then adjust your rearview mirror so that you can use it easily when you're in this position.

Learn the art of self-hypnosis. This can be an instant reliever, according to Dr. Primavera. Just sit in a comfortable chair, close your eyes, and imagine a safe, cozy place. Relax all over until you feel limp and loose from your toes to your head. Then begin breathing evenly and deeply, focusing your mind on the rhythm of your breathing and the sense of feeling sleepy and deeply relaxed. Repeat a soothing message to yourself. "A message as simple as 'make the pain go away' or 'just relax' as a headache begins can be very effective," says Dr. Primavera.

Try the ha-ha-hee-hee-ho-ho remedy. Some people can actually laugh away a headache. A 15- to 30-second laughter prescription can stimulate endorphins, which can eliminate a pain-induced frown and provide a euphoric effect. "Not just a little twitter, but a belly-holding, gut-busting guffaw," says Dale L. Anderson, M.D., an urgent-care physician in Minneapolis and author of health humor books such as *The Orchestra Conductor's Secret to Health and Long Life*.

Here's how he describes it.

• Stand in front of a mirror and give yourself a big, toothy smile.
• Begin laughing—accelerating from a mild ha-ha-ha to all-out guffaws.
• Keep it going until you're laughing at full throttle, holding nothing back.

Act like a kid. "When you feel the pain of a stress headache coming on, ask yourself how an 8- or 10-year-old would deal with this situation," says Joel Goodman, Ed.D., director of The Humor Project in Saratoga Springs, New York. "Sometimes a childlike perspective can be a mature adult coping mechanism."

Mastering the Migraine

The migraine, the most menacing of all headaches, often attacks the entire body. About 24 hours before its arrival, people who are migraine-prone may feel depressed or euphoric, sensitive to light and noise, and prone to excessive yawning.

A migraine can last anywhere from 4 hours to a marathon 72 hours. Many people feel nauseated, have achy, tender neck and scalp muscles, and feel an incessant, throbbing drumbeat on one side of the head. Some may experience an aura, which can cause a temporary loss of speech or visual signals such as flashing lights or a dark blind spot in the center of their vision.

During a migraine, blood vessels leading to the brain expand. As the blood pumps through, a throbbing pain begins. Serotonin, an anti-inflammatory chemical in the brain that is designed to help prevent headaches, is in short supply. But even so, you can fight back with easy exercise if you know the way. Here are some techniques.

Fire up your finger. You can outmuscle a migraine if you master the practice of finger warming. But this is a mind-over-body exercise that takes some concentration and practice.

For headache-free people, the temperature of the index finger is usually around 85°F. But people with migraines usually have finger temperatures in the 70° range—a full 15 degrees or so below "normal." If you can raise your finger temperature to 96°, you can "burn off" a migraine, according to Roger Cady, M.D., director of the Headache Care Center in Springfield, Missouri.

"About 50 percent of people can reduce the frequency of migraines by 50 percent using this type of temperature biofeedback," says Dr. Cady.

If you want to practice, find a quiet place at home where you can either sit or lie down. Make yourself comfortable, but don't cross your arms or legs, says Dr. Cady. Place an oral thermometer on the fleshiest part of your fingertip and secure it with tape. It should read below 95°F when you start. Then:

- Close your eyes.
- Breathe in slowly, stretching your abdomen so that you suck in breath through your nose. Inhale to a count of four.
- Hold your breath for another 4 seconds.
- Exhale through your mouth as you count to eight.

"When you breathe in, say to yourself, 'My hand . . . ,' and as you exhale, say, ' . . . is warm,'" says Dr. Cady. While you're doing this exercise, you should make sure that you clear your mind of interfering thoughts or worries and imagine that the sun is beaming heat into your finger. Continue this exercise for 20 to 30 minutes twice a day.

"The goal is to get the temperature to 96°F at will," Dr. Cady says. "If they have open minds, most people can start to do this." If you do this twice a day to fend off migraines, within 4 or 5 days, you'll begin to see results, he says.

Give yourself a pinch. A pinch in the right spot on the body can banish an approaching migraine, says Michael Blate, an acupressure expert and founder of The G-J Institute in Davie, Florida. "Suffering is the doorbell signaling that it is time to use acupressure," says Blate, author of more than 20 books on natural healing.

For a person who is in good health, acupressure, or the art of applying pressure to ease pain, works fast and effectively, says Blate. But it might not be for everyone. If you're pregnant, using a pacemaker, or taking daily medications for cancer or diabetes, you should check with your physician first, Blate advises.

The easiest method of relieving migraine with acupressure is to press on a spot that's literally right under your nose. Here's what Blate recommends for relief.

- Locate the philtrum—the area of skin between the bottom of your nose and your upper lip.
- Press with the knuckle of your index finger until you feel a small area of discomfort. Massage that spot deeply until the point becomes increasingly tender.
- Stop when you achieve a sense of warmth, perspiration, or clamminess (called an acupressure reaction) across your cheeks or forehead or elsewhere in your body.

The whole process should take only between 30 and 45 seconds, according to Blate. "What happens is that you are changing the energy flow in the body to the head," he says. Blate adds that it not only can help headaches but might give you some side benefits as well. "This point is also useful for nighttime foot aches and certain toothaches," he says.

Say yes to sex. Your partner is in an amorous mood, but you feel a migraine coming on. This is no time to say no, urges Dr. Cady.

Satisfying lovemaking is an exercise that Dr. Cady recommends to stop a migraine dead in its tracks—and it might also conquer a tension headache. Enjoyable sex reduces stress and inspires a sense of well-being, he says. It also may elevate your levels of serotonin.

Supplemental Aid

You can take a preventive approach to headaches with nutritional measures, says Dr. Sheftell. Which supplement you try will depend on which type of headaches you get and what's causing them. Each supplement acts in a different way. You can take supplements in combination without any problems, but your best approach, says Dr. Sheftell, is to try one or two at a time until you find the formula that works for you.

Try Riboflavin for Migraines

In super-high doses, this B vitamin can help ward off a migraine attack by helping the brain cells utilize energy, says Dr. Sheftell.

Pressure Places That Get the Ouch Out

The body has a number of acupressure points that can bring quick relief from tension headaches. Here are two that are recommended by Michael Blate, an acupressure expert and founder of G-J Institute in Davie, Florida.

- With your right hand, squeeze your left thumb as close as possible to the forefinger, forcing a mound of skin to rise between them.
- Place the tip of your right forefinger on that mound and the thumb underneath. Press deeply from above and below, relaxing your left hand. Keep pressing until your right thumb and forefinger discover the tender "ouch" point (called the trigger spot) in the webbing between your thumb and forefinger.
- Massage that trigger spot deeply until the skin becomes tender and you achieve an acupressure reaction, indicated by a feeling of warmth as well as some clamminess or perspiration.
- Continue squeezing while you count slowly to 15.
- Repeat the steps on your opposite hand.

Riboflavin is found in milk. Four glasses will give you the Daily Value of 1.7 milligrams. The doses needed to help prevent migraine are many times higher, however. "All of our patients are put on riboflavin. We start them on 200 milligrams for a week and then bring them up to 400 milligrams," Dr. Sheftell says.

According to Dr. Sheftell, some people experience nausea when they take as much as 400 milligrams. If that happens, you can just return to the 200-milligram dose. It may take some time to get relief, so stick with the supple-

For tension headaches caused by neck and shoulder pain, try this exercise for applying acupressure to the forearm.

- Extend your left hand so that your palm faces the floor.
- Using your right hand, bend your fingers back until you see a crease appear on the top of the left wrist. Release your hand, letting it relax.
- From the position of the crease, measure upward two thumb-widths toward your elbow. Place the middle finger of your right hand in the middle and on top of your left arm and find the space between the two bones.
- Press down with your middle finger, massaging deeply as you count slowly to 15.
- Stop when you feel the warmth or clamminess that signals the acupressure reaction.
- Repeat, using your left hand on your right arm.

ments for 2 to 3 months before you decide whether they have any benefit, says Dr. Sheftell.

Add some magnesium. Another promising migraine fighter is magnesium. This mineral plays a key role in regulating both blood vessel size and the rate at which cells burn energy. Researchers estimate that 50 percent of migraine sufferers are magnesium deficient, says Burton M. Altura, M.D., professor of physiology and medicine at the State University of New York Health Science Center in Brooklyn.

"We believe that everyone should be taking 500 to 600 milligrams of magnesium a day in a combination of diet and supplements," says Dr. Altura. "If people would bring up their total consumption of magnesium, they could reduce the frequency of recurring migraine headaches."

The trouble is, magnesium supplements often cause diarrhea, says Jacqueline Jacques, N.D., a naturopathic doctor and specialist in pain management in Portland, Oregon. This all-too-common side effect is a sign that the supplement is not being absorbed. If you want to get the most from a magnesium supplement and minimize the chance of diarrhea, Dr. Jacques advises taking magnesium glycinate, instead of magnesium oxide or magnesium chloride.

Reap pain relief from fatty acids. Found in high amounts in fish oil and flaxseed oil, omega-3 essential fatty acids provide eicosapentaenoic acid (EPA). In studies, EPA seems to be effective in people who have migraines. Several studies in the 1980s suggested that some people can prevent migraines by taking high doses of fish oil. Take 1,000 to 2,000 milligrams a day in divided doses with meals, says Brent Mathieu, N.D., a naturopathic doctor in Boise, Idaho. The capsules sometimes cause unpleasant, fishy-tasting burping unless you take them with food.

There's also a good chance that you'll get fewer migraines, and less intense ones, if you take 1 to 2 tablespoons of flaxseed oil every day, says Dr. Mathieu. Although you could see an improvement in as little as a few days, 4 to 8 weeks is more typical.

The Headache-Free Lifestyle

You can take steps to reduce headache intrusions into your life, say doctors. "Part of good health is that willingness to nurture yourself," says Dr. Cady. "You have to learn to invest in yourself." That may sound vague and optimistic if you're someone who's prone to headaches, but doctors point out that there are many specific things you can do to "nurture yourself." Here are some of their recommendations.

Don't worry, be happy. Don't overlook the power of smiling as a mental exercise to rid yourself of headaches.

"I don't ever recall a patient coming in with a headache who said, 'Every time I'm terribly happy, I get a headache,'" says Dr. Anderson.

The first step to combat headaches is to boost your mental attitude by improving what Dr. Anderson calls your "smileage." Simply smile more. Think happy thoughts. Along the same lines, do something that makes you happy, he suggests. For some people, that might mean buying a new blouse or shirt. For others, it's sitting by a sunny window, listening to music.

"Anything you do that puts you in a happy place helps your endorphins," says Dr. Anderson. "They also relax muscles," he adds.

Learn to conduct yourself. Ever want to conduct an orchestra? Well, you can—and it might do your head a world of good. To drum out a headache, Dr. Anderson recommends an exercise he calls J'ARM (jog with arms).

First, turn on the radio or put on a favorite CD. Maybe you prefer an energetic Bach classic or a contemporary tune like "Macarena."

"Every time we exercise our arms, our brains say thank you, because by moving our arms, we improve the blood circulation to the brain," Dr. Anderson says. He adds that the life expectancy of orchestra conductors was reported in 1980 to be about 5 years longer than that of the average person.

For your first class in J'ARM school, find a makeshift baton. Simply use whatever is handy—a spoon, a chopstick, or even a handkerchief. As the music starts, raise both arms high and then move them vigorously up and down in exaggerated, enthusiastic conductor motions, keeping time with the music. Sing along. If possible, watch yourself in a mirror during your performance.

If music is not available, you can do this exercise by "playing" a favorite tune in your head and still get the same benefits, says Dr. Anderson. Or just hum to yourself while you conduct your favorite hummable music.

Do some arm twisting. If you're stuck in the office—where wild, J'ARM-style conducting might be frowned upon—you can wrestle with headaches in a more underplayed way. When you've got a spare moment, stand up and let your arms hang relaxed at your sides. Turn your palms inward so they're pressed loosely against your thighs. Inhale deeply, then exhale, and as you do, rotate your arms so that your palms face forward and your thumbs point out. With the next inhalation, again turn your palms toward your thighs. Repeat a few more times, always with a relaxed, effortless motion, says Dr. Cady.

By doing this exercise three to five times daily, you'll begin to dissolve tension in your shoulders, neck, arms, and upper back.

Shrug off pain. If you're weighed down by worry, your back muscles may tighten and your shoulders may slump, triggering a tension headache, says Dr. Cady. To counteract this tension, try a sequence of tensing and relaxing your shoulders.

Stand with your arms hanging at your sides and your shoulders relaxed. Inhale, lifting your shoulders as high as you can. Then exhale, relaxing your shoulders again. On the next breath, lift your shoulders only half as high and then exhale. On your last lift, you should barely raise your shoulders. Repeat this sequence three to five times a day.

Heartburn

Heartburn occurs when stomach acid finds its way up into your esophagus. A little round muscle called the lower esophageal sphincter is the gatekeeper between your throat and your stomach. It's supposed to allow food down and prevent anything from coming back up. But if acid surges past the little muscle and back into the esophagus, you get heartburn. For most people, heartburn is a nuisance, not a serious health threat.

If you're experiencing chronic heartburn, difficulty swallowing, weight loss, weakness, or paleness or if you've had heartburn for 5 years or more and the nature of the heartburn pain suddenly changes (gets worse or better), you should see your doctor.

Turning Down the Burning

For garden-variety heartburn, try these remedies from the experts.

Cultivate new habits. If you're plagued with the symptoms of heartburn, you may want to consider changing your eating habits. Fatty, fried, or high-protein foods, alcohol, and coffee are often the culprits behind heartburn, says Pamela Taylor, N.D., a naturopathic doctor in Moline, Illinois.

Also, pay attention to the final meal of the day, suggests Dr. Taylor. "I tell patients not to eat within 4 hours of their bedtimes and that their last meal of the day should be oriented toward foods such as steamed vegetables, baked or broiled fish, and nonwheat grains such as rice or quinoa," she says.

Take it easy. People who eat quickly and gulp their food often get heartburn, says William Warnock, N.D., a naturopathic doctor in Shelburne, Vermont. He advises people to eat regular meals and, above all, chew food slowly, savoring the smell and taste.

Breathe deeply. This yoga strategy will help douse the fire. Deep breathing makes the diaphragm massage the stomach, and that can relieve heartburn by speeding up digestion, says Richard Miller, Ph.D., a clinical psychologist and cofounder of the International Association of Yoga Therapists in Mill Valley, California.

Most of us just don't breathe deeply enough, says Dr. Miller. When you're taking deep, even breaths, your belly should rise and fall steadily and your shoulders should hardly move at all. If you want to test for this kind of breathing, just put your hand on your belly and watch whether it moves up, down, and out. If you want to stop heartburn, you should check your breathing a number of times during the day to make sure your stomach is rising and falling.

Loosen up. Relief may be as easy as loosening your belt a notch. Wearing pants or skirts that are too tight can create abdominal pressure that can aggravate your heartburn, says M. Michael Wolfe, M.D., chief of gastroenterology at Boston University School of Medicine and Boston Medical Center and coauthor of *Heartburn: Extinguishing the Fire Inside*. When you exercise, for instance, you might want to trade in your tight-fitting spandex pants for a pair of looser-fitting sweats.

Chew gum. Chewing gum stimulates saliva, which contains bicarbonate, a natural antacid, says Dr. Wolfe.

Be upright after meals. Wait at least 3 hours after eating before you lie down. In fact, consider some of these easy activities after a meal, says Stanley Lorber, M.D., former chairman of the gastroenterology department at Temple University School of Medicine in Philadelphia and former team doctor for the Philadelphia 76ers basketball team. They may help you relax and minimize stomach acid.

- Develop a green thumb: Stand at a picnic table to repot some plants.
- Gather your pals for a friendly game of pinochle or Pictionary.
- Join a choir that practices in the evening.
- Take a pleasant after-dinner stroll.

Look to licorice. Deglycyrrhizinated licorice, or DGL, is an excellent herb to soothe heartburn, says Melissa Metcalfe, N.D., a naturopathic doctor in Los Angeles. The typical dose is two 250-milligram capsules taken 20 minutes before mealtime.

Dr. Metcalfe suggests that you suck on the capsules and let them dissolve slowly in your mouth, rather than swallow the DGL with water. You can also get DGL in chewable tablets, which dissolve as you chew them. "You want the licorice to coat the inside of your throat and esophagus to cover those inflamed and irritated tissues," she says.

Use it for 4 weeks and then assess if it's working, she suggests. If it is, your throat should feel less irritated. If not, see your health-care practitioner.

Anti-Heartburn Etiquette Exercises

Some experts believe that heartburn is caused less by what we eat than by how we eat it. Consider this advice from Joyann Kroser, M.D., a gastroenterologist at Presbyterian Medical Center and assistant professor of medicine at the University of Pennsylvania, both in Philadelphia, and Stanley Lorber, M.D., former chairman of the gastroenterology department at Temple University School of Medicine in Philadelphia and former team physician for the Philadelphia 76ers basketball team.

Eat smaller portions. The more food you put in your stomach, the more acid it secretes for digestion. And more acid could mean more heartburn.

Eat slowly. If you eat more slowly, you are likely to eat less. To reduce the gulp factor, get a pair of chopsticks. Unless you're an accomplished user, they'll slow you down.

Chew completely. When your stomach receives partially chewed food, it has to secrete more acid to break it up for digestion. If you become a master masticator, you cut the acid level.

Get at the inflammation. Another healing substance for damaged mucous membranes is glutamine, an amino acid that's available as a nutritional supplement. Dr. Metcalfe frequently recommends it for gastrointestinal disorders whenever inflammation is a problem. "I tell people to take one 500-milligram capsule four times a day until they are feeling better," she says. "Usually, that's about a month."

Kill the bacteria. If bad bacteria—usually *H. pylori*—are the source of your problem, you could consider taking goldenseal, says Dr. Metcalfe. First, though, get a proper diagnosis from your doctor.

For best results, Dr. Metcalfe recommends that you combine a goldenseal supplement with colloidal bismuth, which is the active ingredient in many over-the-counter stomach medications like Extra-Strength Pepto-Bismol. Besides coating the stomach, the bismuth helps the herb adhere to the mucous membranes of the stomach.

Take two or three 400-milligrams capsules of goldenseal daily along with 1 tablespoon of Extra-Strength Pepto-Bismol four times daily, Dr. Metcalfe suggests. "When you take bismuth, be aware that your stools will turn black. It's nothing to worry about." Don't use goldenseal if you are pregnant, however.

Spice up your life. Relief can be as close as your spice rack. Ginger relaxes the smooth muscle along the walls of the esophagus, says Dr. Taylor. "If your digestion is working better, you're less likely to get that reflux, or backwash, of stomach acid," she says. You can take one or two "00" capsules, make a tea from the fresh root or the powder, or eat candied or pickled ginger as it comes from the jar. Ginger tincture is also available. (Dr. Taylor recommends a dose between 15 and 60 drops, repeated as necessary. Add the drops to a little water. If necessary, repeat the 15-drop dose every 15 minutes, up to a total of 60 drops.) If you're using ginger to prevent heartburn, take it 20 minutes before a meal.

Losing Weight the Low-Burn Way

Although people of all shapes and sizes can experience heartburn, it's more common among people who are overweight, especially folks who have their extra pounds around the middle, where they can put pressure on the sphincter muscle. Losing weight around your belly is a great way to stop heartburn.

There's one small problem, though. Exercise, which is usually a crucial part of weight loss, often makes heartburn worse. Why? If you start running, stomach acid sloshes around down there, and it's more likely to splash back up into your esophagus. Before you know it, "feel the burn" has a whole new meaning.

Any gentle weight workout that keeps you vertical and doesn't jostle your stomach contents can be an important weight-loss complement to aerobic exercise, says Dr. Lorber. The more muscle you have, the faster your metabolism. The more quickly your system burns calories, the more easily you'll lose weight. Here are two great exercise options for losing weight without getting burned in the process.

Pedal painlessly. Riding around your block or pedaling in front of the TV is a great way to lose weight without lighting the heartburn fire. Since your tummy doesn't move, your stomach acid stays where it belongs, says Dr. Wolfe.

If you're out of shape, you should build up your biking distance and speed slowly. For the first day, just ride easily for 5 minutes, says Iona Passik, a certified personal trainer, certified master Spinning trainer, and certified group fitness instructor at Chelsea Piers, a fitness center in New York City. (A Spinner is a specialized stationary bicycle that simulates outdoor biking and is used as indoor training for people who bike outdoors.) Each day, add another minute or two, and if you're working out on a stationary bike, increase the resistance a little bit. "Increasing the level of difficulty over time helps you build strength and muscle," Passik says. Work up to three 20-minute sessions a week.

Give yourself a lift. Shape up without burning up by using 5- to 10-pound hand weights, says Dr. Lorber. Doing exercises with light weights should help turn fat into muscle without causing heartburn, he says. For starters, try this lateral lift.

- Sit upright in a straight chair with a dumbbell in each hand, your arms at your sides with your elbows slightly bent and your palms facing your upper thighs).
- Lean forward slightly at the waist, keeping your shoulders back and your back straight.
- Slowly raise your arms out to each side until the dumbbells reach shoulder level. Your arms should be straight and perpendicular to the rest of your body, with your palms facing the floor.
- Hold the position for a second, then slowly lower your arms to the starting position.
- Do a few to start, then gradually work up to two sets of 8 to 12 repetitions.

Hip Pain

The biggest fear among Elvis impersonators may be pelvic bones that howl like a hound dog while getting all shook up on stage.

It's tough to remind anybody of the King if you're hobbled in the hips. But Elvis impersonator Michael Bartle of San Francisco doesn't worry anymore. Why? Because before every performance, he stretches and strengthens his hips with a series of water exercises. "Since I started water workouts before my shows, I am the most limber I've ever been. And I am springier on stage," he says.

The origin of pain in the hip area is often complex. Its most common cause is osteoarthritis, the wearing down of the cartilage cushion between the ball and socket of the joint. But hip pain is sometimes caused by strained (or pulled) muscles. It can also stem from malfunctioning tendons in nearby parts of the body—the lower back, the buttocks, and the upper legs.

If you have severe hip pain, you should consult your doctor before embarking on an exercise program. But for mild cases of hip ache and stiffness, experts recommend an easy-does-it, two-pronged workout strategy that combines stretches for hip flexibility with low-impact strengthening exercises for optimal hip power.

Stretch Those Hips

Stretching—elongating the muscles—helps relax muscles and improve flexibility, says Michael Ciccotti, M.D., orthopedic surgeon and director of sports medicine at the Rothman Institute at Thomas Jefferson University in Philadelphia. Try these.

Make a marriage proposal. The position for this hip flexor stretch, recommended by Thomas Meade, M.D., orthopedic surgeon and medical director of the Allentown Sports Medicine and Human Performance Center in Pennsylvania, looks as if you're about to pop the question to your sweetheart.

- Kneel on your left knee. Bend your right knee, and keep your right foot flat on the floor in front of your body.
- Put your hands on your hips or rest your right hand on your right knee, and let the other hand hang by your side.
- Tighten your abdominal muscles, and lean slightly forward without arching your back. You should feel a stretch in the front of your left thigh. Hold for 20 seconds.
- Repeat three times and then switch legs.

Push away. For variety, try this stretch, recommended by Dr. Meade to relax and improve flexibility in your hip rotator muscles.

- Lie on your back with your knees bent and your feet flat on the floor. To keep your neck from arching, place a pillow under your head.
- Place your left ankle on your right knee.

- Keep your lower back flat on the floor with your left hand on your left thigh. Use your hand to gently push your left knee away from you. You should feel the stretch in the buttocks area.
- Hold this stretch for 20 seconds, then repeat three times.
- Switch legs and repeat.

Rock bottom. To relieve muscle tightness in the buttocks, Meir Schneider, Ph.D., licensed massage therapist, founder of the Center and School for Self-Healing in San

Bo Knows Hips—And Leg Lifts

Former football and baseball player Bo Jackson is proof that it's possible to maintain a healthy body after hip replacement surgery. Jackson was 29 when his hip was replaced, in 1992. "Afterward, it was very important for me to strengthen the muscle groups surrounding my hips," he says.

Now president of HealthSouth Corporation's Sports Medicine Council, based in Birmingham, Alabama, and an actor, Jackson shares his favorite daily hip-strengthening exercises.

- Lie on your back.
- Keeping your right leg straight, bend your left knee and place your foot flat on the floor.
- Raise your right leg 6 inches off the floor and hold for 6 seconds. Repeat 10 times.
- Next, lie on your left side with your left leg slightly bent. Lift your right leg, without turning your knee toward the ceiling, and hold for 6 seconds.
- Repeat 10 times, then do the entire sequence on the other side.

Francisco, and creator of the Meir Schneider Self-Healing Method, offers this hip-rocking stretch from his book *The Handbook of Self-Healing*.

Sit cross-legged on the floor or on an armless chair or stool with your feet flat on the floor. Shift your weight onto your left buttock, then slowly rotate your upper body in a circle over the left buttock (most of the movement will be in the lower back). First, lean forward as far as you can. From that forward position, lean to the left as far as you can. Then rotate backward and finally to the right. Remember to keep your weight on your left side. Try 20 full rotations, then relax and repeat the steps while putting your weight on your right buttock, suggests Dr. Schneider.

Press and please. Sit on a rug or mat so that the soles of your feet touch and your knees are out to both sides, says Dr. Schneider. Be careful to keep your weight evenly distributed on your buttocks. Place one hand on top of

Caution: Don't Be a Hip Hero

Most people can build limber and strong hips through daily stretches and low-sweat leg lifts, says Michael Ciccotti, M.D., orthopedic surgeon and director of sports medicine at the Rothman Institute at Thomas Jefferson University in Philadelphia. But it's important that you don't overdo it. Dr. Ciccotti recommends that you seek immediate medical attention if your hip pain:

- Intensifies during or after exercise
- Radiates from the buttock area down to the leg
- Persists and is not relieved with rest, ice, or over-the-counter pain relievers
- Keeps you up at night
- Keeps you from bearing weight on the hip.

each knee and gently press down, first on your right knee and then the left. Then press both hands down on your knees at the same time. This motion opens the hip joints and stretches your inner-thigh muscles, says Dr. Schneider.

Take your hips for a dip. To fight hip joint stiffness and improve flexibility, water exercises may be ideal, says Jane Katz, Ed.D., professor of health and physical education at John Jay College of Criminal Justice at the City University of New York, world Masters champion swimmer, member of the 1964 U.S. Olympic performance synchronized swimming team, and author of *The New W.E.T. Workout*. Water offers a low-impact workout, takes the weight off your aching hip, and strengthens the muscles around the hip. Here is one of Dr. Katz's favorites.

- Stand in waist- to chest-deep water with your back resting against the pool wall for support.
- Standing on your left leg, cross your right leg in front of your body, grasping your ankle with your left hand. Use your right arm to hold on to the pool edge.
- Slowly bend your left leg. This will stretch the muscles at the hip and the back of your right thigh.
- Slowly straighten up and change legs. Repeat this cycle five times.

A Joint Effort

Add these muscle-toning exercises to your hip flexibility program.

Kick a game-winning field goal. To strengthen the flexor muscles in front of your hip as well as the thigh, hamstring, and buttock muscles, try a little slo-mo air football, says Dr. Ciccotti.

- Stand next to a countertop or sturdy railing and hold on with your left hand.

- While keeping your supporting left leg straight and your foot flat on the floor, raise your right leg as high as you can in front of your body.
- Hold that pose for no longer than a second before letting your leg fall, and slowly swing behind your body as far as possible without straining.
- Hold the position for no more than a second, then swing back to the starting position as if you were kicking a football in slow motion.
- Try 10 swings before switching to the left leg.

By trying to raise your leg higher on each end of the swing, you can increase your range of motion, says Dr. Ciccotti.

Squat down. This do-anywhere exercise helps strengthen the muscles in the fronts of your hips and thighs and your buttocks, says Dr. Meade.

Stand with both feet flat on the floor and hip-width apart. Cross your arms over your chest and face straight ahead, then slowly squat until your thighs are parallel to the floor. Try to keep your torso straight and your knees directly over your toes. Hold the squat for a couple of seconds and then stand up. Try 10 squats twice a day.

Try water wading. To strengthen arthritic hips without jarring pain from pavement, Dr. Katz recommends walking chest-high in H_2O.

Start off slowly by marching in place, raising your knees high as if you were leading the high school band onto the football field at halftime. Slowly pick up speed throughout your workout. Do this for 1 minute and follow it with a minute of rest, then do another minute of stepping, followed by rest. Over time, work up to 3 minutes of continuous exercise.

Intermittent Claudication

Experts have described intermittent claudication as a "heart attack" of the lower leg. It's a painful condition characterized by a cramp in a calf muscle. The cramp, caused by poor circulation, appears during some kinds of exertion when the calf muscles are crying out for more blood and the oxygen that it comes with it. If the cramp is accompanied by chest tightness, it may be an indication of coronary artery disease as well.

"With intermittent claudication, a person will get a deep, painful cramp that feels like it is at the bottom of the calf muscle right next to the bone," says Dan Hamner, M.D., a physiatrist and sports medicine specialist in New York City.

How to stop the cramp? Stop exerting yourself. The cramp will stop pretty quickly once you do, says Dr. Hamner. The only problem is that it will return when you resume exercising. And that poses a painful dilemma, because sometimes the best means of relieving intermittent claudication involves the same activity that triggered the cramp.

"Although intermittent claudication is aggravated by exercise," says Dr. Hamner, "exercise is also the best way to cure it."

To deal with partially blocked blood vessels in your legs, you may be able to create bloodflow bypasses with aerobic activities like walking. When you go for a stroll, sometimes you can stimulate the production of new circulation routes in your legs, according to Dr. Hamner.

Before you add more blocks to your walking regimen, though, Dr. Hamner recommends that you get a thorough checkup and a stress test from your physician. Sometimes, circulation problems in your legs can be an omen of more serious problems elsewhere. About half of the people with intermittent claudication also have coronary arteries that are partially clogged by plaque. "Generally, if you have plaque in your leg arteries—what we call peripheral vascular disease—you need to get a stress test, because your heart may be just as bad," he says.

Walking the Walk

Once your doctor has given you the green light to exercise, here are some exercises that may help alleviate or prevent the leg pain. Don't forget to do a warmup routine before exercising and wear clothing that will keep your legs warm.

Increase your distance. The next time intermittent claudication strikes, slow down until the pain diminishes and then continue your walk at your original rate, says Dr. Hamner. Think of the new blood vessels that you are creating that will deliver the blood to your legs and feet.

"When you start feeling the muscle cramps, try to walk a short distance with the pain before you stop to rest," says Dr. Hamner. "The objective is to extend the distance that you walk. If you always try to increase the distance, you may be able to walk a few hundred yards farther each week."

With 4 weeks of steady walking, Dr. Hamner says, new capillaries will sprout in your legs to help ease the pain caused by the blocked blood vessels.

Head for the hills. Besides gradually building up the distance, Dr. Hamner suggests that you vary your walking routes to include hills as well as flat terrain.

"By varying walking surfaces, you stimulate the formation of new vessels that help blood bypass the blockages," he says. If the pain worsens when you walk uphill, check with your doctor about other possible conditions, such as arthritis of the spine.

Trek on the treadmill. Walking on a shock-absorbing treadmill and climbing on a stair machine can add variety to your workouts, especially during inclement weather, says Dr. Hamner.

Head for the dance floor. You can two-step to keep the pain away by doing the polka, tango, or waltz or even country line dancing, says Dr. Hamner.

"Dancing is a great exercise for this because it requires you to use your calf muscles more," he says. "If you can, try to go up on your toes every now and then while you dance. It will give you a little extra calf work."

Walk in the water. If your calves are really screaming in pain, a few laps of water walking may be in order, says Dr. Hamner.

"I recommend that some people try walking waist-deep in a pool with a water vest on for as long as they can tolerate," he says. "Water aerobics have both cardiovascular and psychological benefits."

Snuff the butts. Nicotine in cigarettes is a vasoconstrictor—meaning it causes your veins and arteries to shrink and constrict. When the pipelines in your legs are already partially blocked, the last thing you need is another impediment to bloodflow, says Frank Fort, M.D., of the Capital Region Vein Centre in Schenectady, New York. "If you're a smoker, you just have to quit. Otherwise, you won't get any better."

Smoking may be the major reason you're having trouble in the first place. It is a major contributor to plaque buildup in the arteries. Cigarette smoke also contains carbon monoxide. Every time you take a puff, carbon monoxide enters your bloodstream, attaches itself to hemoglobin, and robs the blood of its ability to carry oxygen to the muscles.

Nutritional Therapy

Herbs and nutritional supplements may also provide relief. If you've been diagnosed with intermittent claudication, talk to your doctor about trying these remedies.

Open arteries with arginine and magnesium. The amino acid arginine is involved in the production of nitric oxide, a chemical released by the cells lining the artery walls. Nitric oxide allows blood vessels to relax and open up, says Decker Weiss, N.M.D., a naturopathic doctor at the Arizona Heart Institute in Phoenix.

A standard dose is 500 milligrams up to three times a day. If you've been infected by the herpesvirus, though, you should use arginine only with medical supervision, Dr. Weiss says. "In people harboring the virus, high doses of arginine can cause severe outbreaks."

Along with arginine, Dr. Weiss recommends magnesium, an essential mineral. Magnesium is known for its ability to relax the muscles that wrap around blood vessels, so it can help dilate arteries that have been clogged by cholesterol deposits.

You might have a deficiency of magnesium if you are taking drugs, such as diuretics, meant to help heart problems. Some people have deficiencies if they're taking commonly prescribed digitalis heart medications such as digitoxin (Crystodigin) or digoxin (Lanoxin). Signs of magnesium deficiency include muscle weakness, nausea, and irritability.

Most people can safely take up to 350 milligrams of supplemental magnesium, Dr. Weiss says. He recommends it in the form of magnesium orotate or glycinate.

Let B vitamins give you a leg to stand on. Researchers now realize that an amino acid by-product, homocysteine, can harm the insides of blood vessels, setting the stage for the cholesterol deposits that cause intermittent claudication. In one study, researchers were able to reduce high homocysteine levels by using 5 milligrams of folic acid, 400 micrograms of vitamin B_{12}, and 50 milligrams of B_6. "I recommend these B vitamins to all my patients with heart or circulatory problems as part of a high-potency multivitamin or, if they have absorption problems, as injections or under-the-tongue supplements," Dr. Weiss says. This therapy should be done only under a doctor's supervision, he adds.

Get going with gingko. Ginkgo has a reputation for improving circulation in the brain, but it also has body-wide effects that make it useful for all sorts of circulatory problems, including intermittent claudication, Dr. Weiss says. It helps to stimulate growth of new blood vessels and improves the use of oxygen and blood sugar (glucose), the main form of energy for muscle cells.

Ginkgo also helps to reduce the stickiness of clotting components, called platelets, in the blood. When the platelets become less sticky, harmful clots are less likely to form, especially in areas where bloodflow is hindered.

Ginkgo has been tested in several studies of intermittent claudication, and it has worked at least as well as pentoxifylline (Trental), a drug that is commonly prescribed for this problem. Many people in the studies found that when they were taking ginkgo, they could walk much farther without experiencing pain. The supplement also improved bloodflow to the limbs, which was measured using Doppler ultrasound, a noninvasive technique.

Herbalists often recommend 120 milligrams of ginkgo in divided doses of 40 milligrams three times a day. In some studies, however, people have used 160 milligrams a day with good results.

Dr. Weiss's recommendation is lower. He prefers to use a standardized liquid extract of ginkgo, prescribing 20 drops four times a day for at least 6 months.

Act on arteries with antioxidants. People with intermittent claudication usually do better in general if they are taking antioxidant nutrients such as vitamins E and C, which may help prevent the early stages of atherosclerosis (hardening of the arteries), Dr. Weiss says.

Vitamin E has a long history of use for intermittent claudication. In one study, conducted in Sweden, researchers found that they could reduce symptoms if they gave people supplementation with 300 international units (IU) a day.

For smokers, however, supplementation with vitamin E doesn't seem to reduce the symptoms of intermittent claudication. It's quite possible that the vitamin can't entirely overcome the harmful effects that smoking has on your circulatory system, Dr. Weiss says. Breaking the habit comes first.

Dr. Weiss gives many of his patients with atherosclerosis 400 to 800 IU of vitamin E and 1,000 to 3,000 grams of vitamin C a day. Vitamin E helps prevent the oxidation of harmful LDL cholesterol, a first step in cholesterol blockage. Vitamin C regenerates vitamin E and also helps the cells lining the blood vessel walls to produce nitric oxide, which keeps blood vessels open and dilated.

For vitamin E, you should use versions with natural d-alpha-tocopherol and mixed tocopherols, says Dr. Weiss.

Take ginger. "Ginger can be a wonderful addition to a treatment program for intermittent claudication, especially if you also have arthralgia, or pain in your joints," Dr. Weiss says. Like ginkgo, ginger helps keep platelets from getting too sticky, so it keeps your blood flowing smoothly. "It's also a slight vasodilator and a warming herb," Dr. Weiss says, so if you have cold feet, it might provide additional benefits.

Most research studies with ginger use about 1,000 milligrams a day of powdered gingerroot, which is about what you'd get from a ¼-inch slice of fresh root. Ginger is safe to take long-term, Dr. Weiss says.

Perk up with pineapple. Another common food—pineapple—also offers some relief in supplement form. The same ingredient in pineapple that prevents gelatin from setting can help the arteries in your legs stay open, Dr. Weiss says. It's an enzyme called bromelain, which helps keep blood from clotting too readily and may also help existing clots dissolve.

"I might use this if someone with circulatory problems also has had clotting problems in their legs, such as thrombophlebitis," Dr. Weiss says. "Since bromelain also helps to reduce inflammation, I find it's good to use after surgery or injuries," he adds.

Take bromelain between meals; otherwise, it will be used up in the digestion of your meal. A common daily dose used in studies ranges from 60 to 160 milligrams. Dr. Weiss usually recommends much more to his patients—500 milligrams twice a day, as long as needed. With your doctor's supervision, take note of how your body reacts.

Supplement with carnitine. Carnitine, a nutritional supplement, is thought to improve the efficiency of oxygen-starved muscles so that they can do more with less. In other words, carnitine may improve the aerobic metabolism of the muscle.

If you want to try carnitine, Dr. Fort recommends taking 2 grams twice a day orally. You can buy carnitine in health food stores and drugstores. Expect to take the supplement for about a month before you'll start to notice results. Then keep taking the supplement to prevent leg pain. Don't take carnitine without a doctor's guidance, however.

Try red wine. The benefits of red wine have become more evident over the past several years, especially where preventing clots is concerned. Certain elements in red wine seem to inhibit the plaque buildup. One to two glasses of red wine daily is recommended, unless there's a medical or personal reason you shouldn't drink. To be safe, check with your doctor first, says Elliott Badder, M.D., chief of surgery and member of the Vascular Center and Blood Flow Laboratory at Mercy Medical Center in Baltimore.

Irritable Bowel Syndrome

In the scary world of intestinal tracts, the most common ghost—unfortunately—is a mysterious disease that travels under the code name IBS. These three sinister initials are shorthand for irritable bowel syndrome.

People with IBS tend to have alternating constipation and diarrhea, bloating, unformed stools, gas, and sometimes cramps followed by an urgent need to have a bowel movement. As the discomfort goes on, though, the root causes are frustratingly elusive.

IBS is not a disease, and rarely is there any inflammation of the bowel. Doctors who have studied the problem say that it's probably related to stress and food intolerances.

"In my practice, I find that there are two kinds of people who get IBS. First are go-getters who are really stressed; they are hard-wired for stress to stimulate their colons. And then there are the folks who have an intolerance to certain foods," says Leon Hecht, N.D., a naturopathic physician at North Coast Family Health Center in Portsmouth, New Hampshire.

Since the causes are elusive, finding an appropriate remedy can pose a real challenge. Some supplements, however, seem to make the symptoms of IBS more tolerable and possibly less likely to occur, says Dr. Hecht. These treatments—combined with lifestyle and diet changes and stress reduction—may be sufficient for some folks, he says.

Hydrate with water. You need to get enough water, and that may be a good bit more than you're accustomed to drinking. Some people with IBS have small, hard stools that are difficult to pass. By drinking water, they can add soft bulk to the stool and ease its passage through the bowel, says Melissa Metcalfe, N.D., a naturopathic doctor in Los Angeles.

"You should drink eight 12-ounce glasses of water a day, and more if you're an active person," says Dr. Metcalfe.

Get a juicer. Fruit juices are an excellent source of nutrients, but most store-bought juices—especially fortified apple, peach, pear, and prune juices—contain high amounts of sorbitol, a natural sugar that is added to drinks to sweeten them. Sorbitol is hard for the body to absorb and can lead to diarrhea. To get the good effects of fruit juices, without so much sorbitol, you can make your own juices by using a commercial juicer, which can be bought at most department stores.

Minimize milk. Milk isn't much better for people with IBS since many may have lactose intolerance, which can mimic IBS. If in doubt, eliminate dairy products for a while and see if your condition improves.

Bulk up. While you're getting more liquids, also increase the amount of fiber in your diet, Dr. Metcalfe advises. Fiber absorbs water and helps move food and waste more quickly through the gastrointestinal tract. Some excellent sources of fiber are foods like prunes, apples, oat bran, and carrots.

If you need more fiber, you can benefit from a supplement. In a study published in a British medical journal

Some Mint for Movement

Here's a medicine that's good for you, and it tastes good, too. Peppermint has been a popular flavoring agent in candies for centuries, but it has important healing properties as well. It stimulates digestion, relieves gas and bloating, and makes you burp.

The herb's therapeutic qualities are related to its menthol content. Peppermint oil extract contains 50 to 70 percent free menthol, a compound that stimulates bile flow and other gastric secretions in the digestive system. The herb's active oils also have an effect on the sphincter muscle at the lower end of your esophagus. By temporarily changing the behavior of that muscle, peppermint oil extract promotes belching.

Strangely, peppermint also inhibits hunger pangs in the stomach by suppressing peristalsis, the muscular contraction that moves food through the gastrointestinal tract. When the effects of the herb begin to subside, however, the peristaltic movements come back even more strongly.

With more gastric secretions and stronger stomach movements induced by peppermint, food spends less time in your stomach. It is passed along to the small intestine more rapidly, and that means digestion improves.

As a supplement, peppermint oil extract usually comes in capsules. You can also drink peppermint tea.

aptly named *Gut*, 80 patients with irritable bowel syndrome were given either a supplement containing psyllium or a harmless inactive substitute (a placebo). More than 80 percent of the group taking psyllium experienced relief from their constipation, while those in the placebo group noticed no change.

Dr. Metcalfe recommends taking 2 tablespoons daily—in two separate doses—of a fiber/nutritional supplement that contains psyllium husks. Fiber supplements like Metamucil come in a wide range of textures, and some are flavored to make them more palatable. Take them before meals, or take 1 tablespoon in the morning and another before you go to bed. Just make sure that you mix each tablespoon dose with at least two 8-ounce glasses of water, says Dr. Metcalfe.

Calm the colon. Irritable bowel syndrome isn't just irritating; it can be downright painful. When you're having an attack, you can calm your aching colon by taking peppermint oil extract, an herbal medicine long used for digestive problems, says Dr. Hecht. To decrease the severity of your IBS symptoms, you can take it every day.

Peppermint oil extract relaxes the smooth muscles that line the intestines and other internal organs. The herb relieves cramping and calms overactive peristalsis, the muscular contraction that moves food through the gastrointestinal tract. It also helps you belch and relieve gas buildup, according to Dr. Hecht.

In one German study, doctors combined 90 milligrams peppermint oil extract with 50 milligrams caraway oil and gave the mixture to 54 patients with IBS. Others received a placebo. After 4 weeks of taking one capsule before meals, 63 percent of the patients given the oils found that they were pain-free. Only 25 percent of the placebo group noticed any improvement.

Dr. Hecht has found that even peppermint oil extracts alone are effective for some of his patients with IBS. To get the medicine to the intestines, where you need it, look for a peppermint oil capsule or pill that's enteric coated. The coating protects the extract from the acid of the stomach and enables it to release its therapeutic benefits in the small intestine, explains Dr. Hecht.

He suggests a supplement that contains 0.2 milliliters of peppermint oil extract. "Take one capsule between meals three times a day," he says, but he advises that you not take the capsule immediately after a meal.

You may have some discomfort if you take too much peppermint oil since it can cause some burning at the anus. "If that happens, just back off on the dosage and take less," suggests Dr. Hecht.

Be a diet detective. Food intolerance is often a contributing factor to IBS, but the reactions can happen hours after a meal, so people don't always connect what they ate with how they feel, says Dr. Hecht.

Many naturopathic doctors suggest that their patients use the process of elimination to find out what's causing the problem. This is called, logically, an elimination diet. The first step is to cut out the foods that are most likely to be irritants. Many people, for example, have adverse reactions to sugar, wheat, and corn. Milk and other dairy products are common culprits. Chocolate may also be a problem, and a high-carbohydrate diet is involved in 30 to 50 percent of Dr. Hecht's cases. Sometimes, blood testing or allergy testing can provide clues as well, he notes.

For many people, refined sugar is the culprit, says Dr. Hecht. He likens it to a fertilizer for yeast. Although yeast is always present in the body, dietary sugar can lead to an overgrowth in the intestinal tract, resulting in gas, bloating, and pain and triggering cramps and other symptoms of IBS.

Banish the bad bacteria. If bad microorganisms in your intestinal tract start to crowd out the good ones, any problems that you have with food sensitivities or with indigestion may be intensified. One way to combat the problem is to repopulate the gut with good bacteria. Usually, that means that you need to take acidophilus, says Michael

Gazsi, N.D., a naturopathic doctor in Ridgefield, Connecticut.

Acidophilus supplements come in various dosages, depending on the manufacturer, says Dr. Gazsi. Your best bet is to follow the directions on the label and then observe any changes in your condition. A typical dose is one capsule with a meal twice daily.

"If the bowel continues to feel really irritated, I'd back off the dosage a bit or try a different brand," says Dr. Gazsi. "Unfortunately, there's not a lot of quality control with some of these supplements. There's no way of knowing if you're getting enough or too many of the bacteria. You just have to see how you're reacting and adjust accordingly."

Eventually, the good bacteria should re-establish themselves, and you can forgo the acidophilus supplement. Or you can continue taking it. "It's one of those things that you can take indefinitely," says Dr. Gazsi.

Bring on the enzymes. Bacteria aren't the only players in digestion. You also need plenty of digestive enzymes, specialized proteins that break down the food chemically and make it available for use by the body. If enzymes don't do their work properly or are in short supply in the gastrointestinal tract, food passes undigested through the small intestine. As that undigested food reaches the bowel, it may be attacked and consumed by bad bacteria, which in turn causes gas and bloating.

If you're having an irritable bowel problem partly because you lack enough digestive enzymes, you may benefit from taking a supplement to make up for the shortage, says Dr. Gazsi. There are several types on the market. Look for a product that contains plant-derived enzymes, and follow the dosage recommendations on the bottle.

Another way to get your enzymes is to eat more fresh, uncooked vegetables and fruit. You don't get the enzymes from canned, processed, or cooked food since many of the natural plant enzymes are destroyed by cooking and processing, according to Dr. Gazsi.

"You don't want to eat too much raw food all at once, though," he says. "Some people try to change their diets too quickly, which may make their irritable bowels even worse."

Coat and soothe. Although the exact cause of IBS isn't known, herbs that are generally soothing and healing to the digestive tract can be helpful. These herbs, known as demulcents, have the ability to coat mucous membranes.

By direct contact, the demulcents help relieve inflammation and are therefore very soothing, explains Pamela Taylor, N.D., a naturopathic doctor in Moline, Illinois.

A good example is slippery elm. When a dose of 1 to 2 tablespoons of liquid extract is dissolved in water or juice or added to a cooked cereal as a demulcent, it forms a soothing coating that bathes the intestinal walls. "Demulcents such as slippery elm also have a wound-healing effect," she adds.

Supplement combinations of demulcent herbs usually include slippery elm, marshmallow root, echinacea, goldenseal, and geranium. This combination is commonly known as Robert's Formula and is often recommended by naturopathic physicians, says Dr. Taylor.

Kidney Stones

The pain of passing a kidney stone has been compared to the pain of childbirth. With childbirth, there's a sweet reward. With a kidney stone, there's nothing but the production of a granular object.

Men are more likely than women to get calcium stones, and genes play a role as well. Because of that genetic factor, if your parents or grandparents had kidney stones, you're at higher risk for getting them yourself.

Some people have a tendency to excrete high levels of calcium oxalate and calcium phosphate. If all goes well, you get rid of these calcium salts every time you urinate. But sometimes, however, the salts hang around the kidneys like bad leftovers. Eighty percent of all kidney stones are composed of these calcium salts.

The stones can't be ignored, and there's no way to treat them yourself. If you have a stone, you may have severe pain, blood in the urine, and fever. Any of these symptoms should tell you to see a doctor as soon as possible. "It can be a medical emergency. The pain can be excruciating," says Anne McClenon, N.D., a naturopathic doctor at the Compass Family Health Center in Plymouth, Massachusetts.

Sometimes a small stone will pass on its own—with that childbirth-type pain mentioned earlier. If you have a stone that's too big to pass, your doctor will probably recommend an ultrasound procedure that will break it up without surgery.

There are a few strategies and supplements that might help you avoid forming another kidney stone from calcium salts. First, however, you should see your doctor and have a blood test and chemical analysis of your urine and stones to determine if calcium is really your problem. There are other types of stones, and these can form because of a urinary tract infection, gout, or a hereditary kidney disorder.

Stopping Stones

If you're prone to getting calcium stones, here are some tactics and some supplements to help prevent them.

Bypass oxalates. Diet is important if you're trying to avoid kidney stones. Stay away from foods such as spinach, beans, parsley, tea, and coffee. Although some of these items are normally thought of as healthy foods, they are rich in oxalates, says Dr. McClenon. If you have a problem turning oxalates into a form that your body can use, they remain in your urine. "They may precipitate as a stone," she says.

Drink up. Water, that is. It's a simple bit of advice, but it makes a lot of sense when you consider that stones come from dissolved solids, says Leon Hecht, N.D., a naturopathic doctor at North Coast Family Health in Portsmouth, New Hampshire.

It's similar to the rationale behind adding more and more water to soup that's too salty. The objective is to keep the saltwater solution in the kidneys extremely diluted so that a concentration of stone-forming salts doesn't get stuck there. Water causes the concentration of chemicals in the urine to decrease, making them more soluble and less likely to form stones.

Drink at least 8 to 10 full 12-ounce glasses of water each day. Not juice or soda or milk—just water, says Dr. Hecht. (Salt and sugar can raise the level of calcium in your urine.) "You should drink enough so that you're urinating every couple of hours," he adds.

Contain condiment consumption. You should reduce your sodium intake to 2 to 3 grams per day, according to the National Kidney Foundation. Avoid table salt and condiments high in sodium, such as ketchup and mustard. Reduce consumption of processed and pickled foods, luncheon meats, and snack foods such as chips and pretzels.

Beware of stomach antacids. Some antacids are enormously high in calcium, warns Peter D. Fugelso, M.D., medical director of the kidney stone department at the Hospital of the Good Samaritan and clinical professor of urology at the University of Southern California, both in Los Angeles. If you've had a calcium stone and if you need to take an antacid, check the ingredients listed on the side of the box and make sure the antacid is not calcium-based. If it is, choose another brand.

Stonewall with magnesium. Having high levels of calcium oxalate and calcium phosphate in your urine isn't a problem as long at you excrete those salts. For that to happen efficiently, they need to hook up in the urine with other essential chemicals. Otherwise, they'll clump together, form crystals, and precipitate out like sugar settling to the bottom of a glass of iced tea.

That's where magnesium comes in. It binds with the calcium salts so they stay dissolved in the urine.

Magnesium is a regulator of calcium, says Michael Gazsi, N.D., a naturopathic doctor in Ridgefield, Connecticut. "You excrete it rather than have it settle out in the kidney," he explains. "If you keep the magnesium ratio in the urine high, there's less chance of forming a stone."

If you have a predisposition to calcium stones, Dr. Gazsi suggests that you take 500 to 1,000 milligrams of magnesium a day. "It's the single best thing you can do to prevent these types of stones," he says.

Boost protection with B$_6$. For added insurance, you can take a vitamin B$_6$ supplement since B$_6$ reduces the production of oxalate, says Dr. Hecht.

He recommends taking 25 to 50 milligrams of vitamin B$_6$ daily, along with a magnesium supplement. "Magnesium alone decreases the likelihood of kidney stones, but when you put it with vitamin B$_6$, it has an even greater effect," he says.

Keep your Cs low. Vitamin C is good for protecting your cells and boosting immunity, but high doses may be a problem for people with a tendency toward kidney stones, says Dr. McClenon. That's because one by-product of vitamin C is oxalate.

While this doesn't mean that you should avoid vitamin C entirely, it's probably a good idea to limit your dosage to no more than 2,000 milligrams a day, says Dr. McClenon.

Some research suggests, however, that for the average person, vitamin C does not promote kidney stones. It may even have a mild protective effect, according to Alan Gaby, M.D., professor of nutrition at Bastyr University in Bothell, Washington.

Leg Pain

It's a wonder our legs don't hurt all the time. Ever since you learned to get up and walk around on them, your legs have been doing a lot of the heavy work for the rest of your body. Aside from carrying your body weight whenever you're upright, your legs—and the veins and muscles that make up your legs—also absorb hundreds of foot-pounds of pressure with every step you take.

Subjected to a lifetime of nonstop labor, your legs are bound to complain once in a while. Usually, it will be after you walked around too much at the mall, stood in line too long at Walt Disney World, or spent 3 hours crammed into the coach section of an airliner.

Leg pain can be caused by a pinched nerve in the back (sciatica) or from joint ailments like osteoarthritis. But if it's related to the circulatory system, the most likely culprits are varicose veins, phlebitis, and arteriosclerosis (plaque buildup) in the arteries of the legs, which leads to a condition known as intermittent claudication. See also "Intermittent Claudication."

Varicose Veins

Genetics plays a big role in why you have varicose veins. If your mother or a grandparent had them, you may have inherited the tendency. You may also get varicose veins, however, if you sit or stand in one position for long periods or are overweight.

The problem lies not so much with the veins but with the valves in the veins that prevent blood from flowing back into the legs. Because it's a liquid, blood naturally wants to run downhill. It's only the force of your heart pumping and the muscles in your legs that keep it moving against gravity. When you move your legs, your muscles in the calf massage the veins and "milk" the blood upward. Doctors refer to this mechanism as the calf pump.

The valves in the vein keep the blood from dripping back. But if they aren't closing properly, blood pools up into little lakes, and the veins expand with the added volume.

Initially, all you may get are spider veins—faint red lines along the skin surface—but eventually, these varicosities may grow in size. When that happens, you get a dull, generalized ache in the legs and sometimes a throbbing pain.

Use gravity. When your legs feel heavy and achy, put up your feet and create a slope that will make it easier for blood to flow back toward your heart, says Normand Miller, M.D., at the Vascular Center and Blood Flow Laboratory at Mercy Medical Center in Baltimore.

Lie on the floor and put your feet up on the couch, or tilt back in a recliner.

"Putting your legs up helps to empty the venous system. It gets that stagnant blood out of there," says Dr. Miller. "Just a few minutes of this can help you feel better."

For sleeping at night, you can place bricks or a couple

of blocks of wood under the posts at the foot of the bed, says Frank Fort, M.D., of the Capital Region Vein Centre in Schenectady, New York. "It doesn't have to be a steep decline. Two to 4 inches is usually enough."

Shake a leg. The worst thing for your varicose veins is inactivity, says Dr. Fort. Don't spend all day sitting in that chair or lying on the couch. Take a walk, pedal an exercise bike, or do the tango. You have to move around.

"Exercise activates the calf pump and helps build strength in the venous system," he says. "Exercise can only help."

Apply pressure. When your veins are weak and expand easily, you can give them added support by wearing pressure stockings. These elastic stockings put pressure on your tissues and compress areas of stagnant blood in your legs.

"The idea is to squeeze those lakes and turn them into rivers," says Dr. Miller. You can buy pressure stockings in most drugstores and medical supply stores. A general support hose may be enough if your only complaint is fatigue in the legs.

"For most people, a light-support knee-high stocking is enough," he says. "But if a woman chooses to wear support panty hose, that's fine, too."

Note: Wear these stockings only during the day. Take them off at night, but keep your legs elevated for support while you are sleeping.

Phlebitis

There are two types of phlebitis: clotting in the superficial veins of the leg and deep-vein thrombosis, or clotting in the main channels that return blood to the heart.

You're more likely to get superficial phlebitis if you have varicose veins, although men sometimes develop it without a lot of symptoms of varicose veins, says Dr. Fort.

Something as simple as a blow, mosquito bite, or bee sting to the leg can cause a vein to distend or expand.

When that happens, blood no longer flows straight and smoothly but more slowly and turbulently. Instead of a river, you end up with a small lake of blood. Sometimes it congeals, hardens, and forms a clot. Inflammation may set in, says Dr. Fort. You may notice a redness and feel a hard cord or bulge beneath the skin, he explains.

"When you press on it, it hurts. It can be real sensitive to the touch," he says. "It may also hurt when you're walking or moving your leg." Even though it can reach the diameter of a garden hose, a superficial clot is not life threatening, he says. Rarely does it travel far along the course of the affected vein.

If you have a tendency to form superficial clots, you may be in danger of having deep-vein thrombosis, which forms a painful type of clot that may move to your lungs. And that is a much more serious matter, says Dr. Fort. That's why you want to get checked out by a doctor whenever you experience leg symptoms such as unusual swelling or pain. The doctor can determine which type of clot you might have and can treat you accordingly.

Otherwise, you can help ease the pain of phlebitis yourself with these measures.

Take a break. If you know you're prone to any type of phlebitis, take precautions. Sitting in one place too long will definitely put you at risk, says Dr. Miller.

When you're traveling for long periods, exercise your legs frequently. If you're riding in a car, make sure to stop every 2 hours and walk for 3 to 4 minutes. On a cross-country flight, get up and walk down the aisle every hour or so.

Tap your feet. Even while you're seated, it's a good idea to keep the blood moving, rather than let it pool in your legs. Lift up on the balls of your feet and flex your calf muscles, says Dr. Fort.

What this does is activate the calf pump in the leg. As you flex the muscle, you squeeze the veins and pump the venous, unoxygenated blood from your legs.

"If you can't get up and walk around, you want to at least keep your feet moving," he says.

Leg Cramps

Baseball players coined the term *charley horse* more than 100 years ago for the cramps they got in their tired, overworked leg muscles.

Whether you're running the bases or lying in bed, nerves send signals to the muscles to tell them when to contract and relax. When these signals get scrambled, the muscle responds by cramping.

What mixes up the messages? The first suspected cause is a mineral imbalance, says Jacqueline Jacques, N.D., a naturopathic doctor and specialist in pain management in Portland, Oregon. That's not the only possibility, though. Cramps can also be caused by strenuous exercise, excessive salt loss from sweating, or sitting or standing too long.

When you get a cramp, stretch and gently massage the muscle immediately. This should relax the muscle and provide you with some much-needed relief. If you find that you're having muscle cramps every night, your doctor is likely to prescribe quinine, but only for a limited time. This often-used treatment for leg cramps can quickly build to toxic levels in the blood and can cause nausea, vomiting, ringing in the ears (tinnitus), and deafness. It can even damage your eyesight.

There are safer ways to eliminate that knot of pain in your muscles, such as the following.

Pinch away pain. Ready for instant relief? Try this acupressure technique. Grab your upper lip between your thumb and index finger, and squeeze for about 30 seconds.

Get a Leg Up

Here are some exercises to do a few times a day to activate the calf pump and improve vein circulation in the
legs. Doing the exercises while lying down enables you to
take advantage of gravity. If you have varicose veins,
you should do these exercises at least twice a day, but
three or four times a day if possible, says Frank Fort,
M.D., of the Capital Region Vein Centre in Schenectady,
New York.

First, lie on your back with your legs straight. Then
lift your legs up and rest them on a box, the edge of a
chair, or several piled-up pillows so that your legs are
straight and at a 45-degree angle, says Dr. Fort. Your
legs should contact the box or chair at mid-calf, leaving
your feet free to move.

The following three exercises should all be done
from this position.

- Flex your toes forward and then backward at a
  comfortable pace. Repeat this back-and-forth motion for 30 seconds.
- Moving your feet at the ankle, draw circles in the
  air with your feet. Draw five circles clockwise,
  then five circles counterclockwise.
- Move your feet back and forth as a way of flexing
  your calf muscles. Alternate so that your right foot
  is flexed while your left foot is pointed, then switch.
  Flex 10 times in a period of about 30 seconds.

"It's hard to believe, but it works great," says Patrice
Morency, a sports injury management specialist in Portland, Oregon, who works with Olympic hopefuls. Although there's no definite explanation for *why* acupressure

works, it's a pain-relief technique many athletes have found to be effective.

Let your fingers do the massaging. You can use the direct approach, too: Grab the cramping muscle tightly, and push your fingertips deep into the cramp for about 10 to 15 seconds, then release. You can repeat as often as necessary to relieve the cramp, says Morency.

Contract and relax. Contracting any muscle that opposes a cramping muscle forces the cramped one to relax, says Morency. When you suffer a severe leg cramp in the calf muscle, for example, flex your shin muscle (which opposes your calf muscle) by pulling your toes toward your knee.

Better yet, while you're pulling your toes up, have a friend gently press the top of your foot the other way to provide resistance, says Morency. That maxes out the tension on your shin muscle, which should cause the cramped calf to release.

Stretch toward comfort. After the cramp is gone, stretch out the muscle—but begin slowly and without bouncing on it, says Andy Clary, head trainer for the University of Miami football team in Coral Gables, Florida. Here's a stretch that will ease the hamstring, which lies under the thigh, almost behind the knee: To begin, sit down on the floor and extend the leg. Then reach out and gently pull your toes toward your knee. That applies pressure over the belly of the hamstring muscle, stretching it comfortably. "You simply want to elongate the muscle," says sports injuries specialist Craig Hersh, M.D., of the Sports Medicine Center in Fort Lee, New Jersey.

Mix in magnesium. If you're getting a nightly wake-up call from your leg muscles, you probably need to get more magnesium and calcium, says Mark Stengler, N.D., a naturopathic doctor in Beaverton, Oregon, and author of *The Natural Physician: Your Health Guide for Common Ail-*

ments. Both of these minerals are involved in relaxing nerve impulses and regulating muscle activity. Calcium is needed to contract the muscle, and magnesium is needed to relax it. An imbalance in this dynamic duo can irritate and confuse the muscle.

Start with a dose of 250 milligrams of magnesium glycinate or chelated magnesium twice a day, says Dr. Jacques. These amino acid–based mineral supplements are easier to absorb than magnesium oxide. The more you absorb, the less likely it is that you'll have diarrhea, a common problem with magnesium supplements.

Dr. Jacques is definitely not an advocate of magnesium oxide supplements. "Magnesium oxide is basically a rock," she says. "The reason it causes diarrhea is that it stays in the gut. We even see it occasionally on x-rays, where it shows up like little bone chips."

To help relieve cramps that interrupt your nightly Zzzs, take your second dose of magnesium right before you go to bed. If you don't get relief in 3 to 5 days, increase the dose to 500 milligrams twice a day, says Dr. Jacques. Stay at that level for another week to allow the tissue levels of the mineral to build up.

Take time for calcium. If cramps are still a problem at that dosage of magnesium, it's time to add 500 milligrams of calcium to the regimen. The average adult absorbs only about 30 percent of the calcium consumed.

To maximize absorption, Dr. Jacques gives her patients calcium citrate instead of calcium carbonate, the form commonly found in antacid tablets. It helps to take it with a glass of milk since vitamin D is necessary for calcium absorption. If you are unable to drink milk, you can take a calcium supplement that contains vitamin D.

Do the math. If you're taking both calcium and magnesium, keep in mind that they work best when they are taken in certain ratios. The two ratios recommended by naturopathic doctors are either equal doses of calcium and magnesium or twice as much calcium as magnesium. "A lot of it is a guessing game, particularly with something like leg cramps," says Dr. Jacques. "You have to find out what ratio works best for you."

Try the one-to-one ratio first, taking 500 milligrams of calcium and 500 milligrams of magnesium twice a day, Dr. Jacques says. If that doesn't give you the results you want, shift the ratio to 2:1 by reducing the magnesium to 250 milligrams.

Take E and see. Some patients with nighttime cramping have success with vitamin E, says Dr. Stengler. Although it has had mixed results in clinical trials, early studies suggest that you'll improve arterial bloodflow and reduce leg cramping at night if you take vitamin E.

In one of the largest studies, 123 of 125 people who suffered from nighttime leg and foot cramps reported complete relief after taking vitamin E supplements. To see if it works for you, take 400 to 800 international units (IU) a day, says Dr. Jacques.

Provide your muscles with potassium. Potassium is another mineral that helps regulate muscle contraction, says Dr. Stengler. Deficiencies of this crucial electrolyte aren't normally a problem if you eat a variety of fruits and vegetables. If you change your diet drastically, however, you might become deficient. This is a potential problem if you go on one of the high-protein weight-loss diets that some experts advocate.

"When people go on high-protein diets, they begin to develop leg cramps. I see it repeatedly," says Dr. Jacques. She believes that such diets are related to potassium deficiency.

When protein makes up more than 30 percent of your daily calories, potassium levels may fall far short of the DV of 3,500 milligrams, according to Dr. Jacques. If you're eating eight or nine servings of fruits and vegetables, you'll get enough potassium to meet the DV, but the shift to a high-protein diet makes this significantly more of a challenge.

Cramps are more prevalent when you first start a high-protein diet, Dr. Jacques has observed. After a few months, they normally disappear on their own. To make them go away sooner, you can take one 99-milligram tablet of potassium a day, she suggests. This doesn't amount to much more than a bite or two of banana, but it can make your legs feel better, she says.

A word of caution, though: Don't take more than one tablet. It's easy to get too much potassium this way, which can upset the balance of other minerals in your body and cause heart and kidney problems. That's why Food and Drug Administration regulations don't allow more than 99 milligrams per tablet in over-the-counter supplements.

Loosen your legs with trace minerals. When you get leg cramps, the first suspects are naturally the big minerals that we've already discussed—calcium, magnesium, and potassium. But maybe those cramps are due to an imbalance of trace minerals, especially if the pain is triggered by overexertion, says Dr. Jacques. "Muscle and nerve function are electrical, and we need the right mix of minerals for that to happen. There are a lot of little players in there."

You can deplete levels of trace minerals as you perspire. Electrolyte drinks work well to help restore these depleted minerals. You can also take a trace mineral supplement that contains copper, manganese, zinc, selenium, and chromium, says Dr. Jacques.

Although trace mineral supplements vary in content, don't exceed the dosage guidelines on the bottle, she says. "Trace minerals should be taken in small doses because that's how they are found in your body. More is not better."

If you get leg cramps when you walk, see your doctor to rule out other conditions such as intermittent claudication, which is caused by poor bloodflow to the legs.

Soothe spasms with herbs. Herbal extracts offer a natural way to soothe and relax spastic muscles. One of the most valuable is black cohosh, says Dr. Stengler. Also known as black snakeroot and bugbane, black cohosh root contains active substances called triterpene glycosides, antispasmodics that act as natural muscle relaxants.

When muscles seize up with pain, take a 500-milligram capsule of the root powder or 30 to 60 drops of tincture in warm water every 1 to 2 hours.

For acute cramps, two or three doses should be sufficient for a therapeutic effect, says Dr. Stengler. Don't use black cohosh during pregnancy, though, or for more than 6 months at a time.

Bilberry contains chemicals called anthocyanins, a type of flavonoids that have muscle-relaxant properties. Bilberry also helps to improve circulation in the extremities. To reduce muscle cramping, three times a day take 80 milligrams of an extract standardized to contain 25 percent anthocyanidin. You should take it for at least a couple of months, but you can continue indefinitely if necessary, says Dr. Stengler.

"Ginkgo is also useful since it improves circulation through the extremities by dilating the arteries that feed the leg tissue," he says. When cramps are a problem, Dr. Stengler gives patients 60 milligrams three times a day of an extract containing 24 percent ginkgoflavoglycosides and 6 percent terpenelactones. If you have circulation problems, you can probably use ginkgo on a long-term basis.

Muscle Soreness

In a classic episode of the venerable *I Love Lucy*, Lucy had a chance to meet a slew of British royalty, including the Queen. In conscientious preparation, Lucy set out to learn a perfect curtsy. After an afternoon's practice—half deep-knee bends and half forward lunges—her over-worked muscles were frozen in curtsy position. When the moment finally came, Lucy had to be toted like a doubled-up curtsy doll to meet Her Majesty.

Very funny—right?

If you recall experiencing that kind of overstrained pain, you probably found it no laughing matter.

One culprit, whether you're practicing curtsies or working out, is lactic acid. As it builds up in muscles, lactic acid creates the soreness that we associate with overexertion. If your body's in good working order, how-ever, it quickly purges this waste product, usually within an hour.

Soreness that comes a day or two after you exercise has a different source. The delayed ache is caused by tiny tears in the muscle that become inflamed. Fitness experts call it delayed-onset muscle soreness, but you probably know it as plain old pain. It's a signal from your body to slow down and take a rest. It's also part of the recovery process that actually results in stronger muscles.

You can prevent sore muscles by warming up before you exercise and cooling down afterward, advises Jacob Schor, N.D., a naturopathic doctor in Denver and president of the Colorado Association of Naturopathic Doctors. Include at least a few minutes of movement with each of the major muscle groups—the calves, thighs, hips, back, abdomen, chest, and arms.

Get Fast Relief

For the immediate pain, try these remedies.

Have an ice day. You may be able to recover from muscle pain more quickly by icing the muscles that are complaining, says William J. Evans, Ph.D., director of the nutrition, metabolism, and exercise laboratory at the University of Arkansas for Medical Sciences in Little Rock. "Your muscles swell somewhat when you damage them from overuse. Ice can help to reduce the inflammation." Wrap a frozen ice pack in a thin towel and place it on the affected area for no more than 20 minutes each hour. You can repeat as often as necessary until the area is no longer sore. If an ice pack isn't handy, you can use a bag of frozen peas wrapped in a towel instead.

Turn up the heat. When the aches and pains are particularly bad the day after you've exercised hard, take a warm bath, says Priscilla Clarkson, Ph.D., professor and associate dean in the department of exercise science at the University of Massachusetts School of Public Health and Health Sciences in Amherst. You can soak for as long as you like, she says. "The warm water helps your muscles relax and promotes circulation, which will have a soothing effect. The pain will come back 15 minutes or so after you get out, but it still makes for a nice break."

Ask for acetaminophen. Other over-the-counter medications will probably reduce pain, but acetaminophen (Tylenol) is the best choice for muscle pain, says Dr. Evans. Why? Other possible painkillers on the pharmacy shelf—aspirin, ibuprofen (Advil), ketoprofen (Orudis KT), and naproxen (Aleve)—all share a single drawback. These anti-inflammatory drugs block your body's production of chemicals that cause swelling and pain, but in so doing they interfere with your body's muscle-repair process.

Acetaminophen, on the other hand, blocks pain impulses within the brain itself, allowing the muscle-repair process to proceed normally, says Dr. Evans. It's also the pain reliever that causes the fewest side effects when taken in normal amounts. Just make sure to follow the directions on the label, and never take more than 12 of the 325-milligram pills in a single day.

Get home-style help. If you prefer a drug-free remedy, take ginger, says Dr. Schor. "It's kind of like a home-style ibuprofen." Ginger is well-known for its anti-inflammatory properties and contains an enzyme that can break down protein, says Dr. Schor.

Ginger also contains various antioxidants, which help neutralize the free-roaming, unstable molecules called free radicals that play a role in causing inflammation. To use ginger as a supplement, take it in tincture or capsule form. If you're in acute pain, take six 500-milligram capsules extract per day of the concentrated, says Dr. Schor.

Do some damage control. Even before your muscles seize up, you can get a jump on the healing process with bromelain, an enzyme derived from pineapple, says Dr.

Schor. "If I know I'm going to be sore tomorrow—that I'm not going to want to get out of bed in the morning—I take bromelain."

Like the cleanup crew the morning after a big bash, bromelain goes in and picks up all the debris floating around your damaged muscle. When you overwork a muscle enough to cause pain, bits of muscle fiber actually break off. These tiny scraps of protein may clog the muscle and cause pain and inflammation. The body has to clean house.

Because it's an enzyme, bromelain helps by breaking down these proteins and digesting them. Once the waste products are eliminated, pain and stiffness go away, says Dr. Schor.

To speed up your muscle-repair work, take 500 milligrams of bromelain three times a day between meals until the pain goes away, says Dr. Schor. If you take it with meals, bromelain's protein-digesting powers will work on your food, not on the muscle debris that's prompting your pain and inflammation.

Be sure to check the product label to make sure that it specifies a strength of 1,800 to 2,400 milk-clotting units (mcu). "When it's not on the label, it makes me suspicious," cautions Dr. Schor. "The company may not know what it's doing, or it may have a very weak product and not want anyone to know." Bromelain is also sometimes measured in gelatin-dissolving units (gdu). Look for a range of 1,080 to 1,440 gdu.

Power up with antioxidants. Because your muscles produce more free radicals when you exercise, you should take supplements of vitamins C and E, says Mark Stengler, N.D., a naturopathic doctor and author of *The Natural Physician: Your Health Guide for Common Ailments.* A healthy supply of these nutrients will help minimize pain the day after your workout and will speed the healing process as your body rebuilds its muscle tissue.

Vitamin C is also needed to help make collagen, the "glue" that holds muscle cells together. Following an injury, even a minor one like a sore muscle, the body needs to make more collagen to repair the damaged tissue. Vitamin E helps reduce muscle soreness, prevent cellular damage, and repair muscle tissue.

To get your dose of pain prevention, take 2,000 milligrams of vitamin C in divided doses each day, along with 400 international units of vitamin E, says Dr. Stengler.

Train without pain. Siberian ginseng, an herb used by Russian cosmonauts and Asian Olympic athletes, can help you train for your next marathon—or your next curtsy before the Queen. "It's classified as an adaptogen, meaning that it helps the body adapt and recover from physical stress," says Dr. Stengler.

The herb helps the adrenal glands produce more stress hormones. Those stress hormones, in turn, help your body recover more quickly from the effects of strenuous or muscle-straining exercise.

The name Siberian ginseng is really a misnomer since the plant is not even in the same genus as true ginseng. Still, its stimulant and tonic effects are similar to those of true ginseng. Clinical studies suggest that ginseng can improve athletic performance, says James A. Duke, Ph.D., botanical consultant, former ethnobotanist with the U.S. Department of Agriculture who specializes in medicinal plants, and author of *The Green Pharmacy*. He notes that you may have to take Siberian ginseng regularly for a month before it begins to yield benefits.

In your quest for peak performance, take 250 milligrams of Siberian ginseng three times a day, says Dr. Stengler. While you are training, take the ginseng for 4 weeks, then take a break for 1 week. Look for a standardized extract containing 0.4 percent eleutherosides.

Relieving Muscle Cramps

Too many hours raking leaves or weeding the flower bed—even marathon hours spent pressing the gas pedal on a long drive to the vacation cottage—can surface hours later as clenching muscle contractions. Although legs are the most common targets, cramps also stalk our feet, thighs, backs, shoulders, and necks.

"Any muscle that's used repeatedly is likely to get fatigued and more likely to cramp," explains John Cianca, M.D., assistant professor of physical medicine and rehabilitation and director of the sports and human performance medicine program at Baylor College of Medicine in Houston. "It just so happens that since we are on our feet all day long, the calf muscles are usually the first to go."

Any muscle that is overstretched or strained can react by cramping. Or you may get that reaction if you hit a muscle directly—by banging your thigh into the corner of the kitchen table, for instance. Sudden changes in temperature also can trigger cramps, says Dr. Cianca.

Although cramps can be plenty painful, they usually subside within a few minutes. To deal with them, you may want to begin with ice and massage, but the full complement of treatment and prevention strategies includes stretching and strengthening exercises, Dr. Cianca explains.

Calf Cramps

Almost as scary as nightmares, painful calf cramps jolt many of us innocent and unsuspecting souls from a deep sleep, say doctors.

These nocturnal nemeses can strike anyone at any age,

but we're more likely to get nighttime cramps as we get older, according to experts.

Here are some quick remedies provided by Dr. Cianca to reduce the pain of a calf cramp and return you to a sound sleep. These techniques also work for daytime calf cramps.

Take a stand. What sounds simple is also effective. When a nighttime cramp sets your calf throbbing, get up and stand tall. Raise your hands straight over your head, and hold this pose for at least 10 seconds. This ministretch reverses the direction of the muscle contraction.

Grab a towel or a T-shirt. If leg cramps have wakened you before, be as prepared as the Boy Scouts for the next assault. Keep a bath towel, a T-shirt, or a piece of rope within reach of your bedside.

When a muscle cramp hits at 3:00 A.M., loop the cloth or rope around the arch of your foot. You can lie on your back or your side, but keep the cramped leg straight and bend your other knee slightly. Slowly pull both ends of the towel or rope toward your chest, tugging the top of your foot toward your shinbone. Hold that stretch for 20 to 30 seconds and repeat a few times until the cramp vanishes into the night.

Massage the muscle. One effective cramp buster is a 5-minute massage on the calf muscle. "Work the calf muscle up and down with the heel of your hand for about 5 minutes or until it feels good," says Dr. Cianca.

Take a slow stroll. You can also try to walk off the calf cramp. With each step forward, gently stretch your toes up toward your shin to lengthen the cramped muscle.

Tight Feet

Second only to the calves, your toes and feet are other hot spots for muscle cramps. Doctors offer these cramp calmers.

Roll in the relief. When a cramp puts your foot in a spasm, hobble over to the kitchen for relief. Kick off your shoe and grab a wooden rolling pin from the drawer. (An empty soda or wine bottle, tennis ball, or golf ball will also do the trick.)

Plant the arch of your cramping foot on top of the rolling pin and hold on to a chair or table for stability. Slowly move the bottom of your foot back and forth over the rolling pin for a few minutes. Most of your weight should be on your good foot, but try putting some weight on the painful foot. "You're helping to get the muscles more relaxed," says Leonard A. Levy, D.P.M., professor of podiatric medicine and past president of the California College of Podiatric Medicine in San Francisco.

Do some lifts. Try the following two exercises the next time your toes or feet get crabby, says Dan Hamner, M.D., a physiatrist and sports medicine specialist in New York City.

First, stand so the weight of your body is on your heels and your toes are slightly off the floor, supporting yourself by holding on to a chair or table. Maintain that pose for at least 5 seconds, feeling the stretch in your ankles and calves. Lower your toes until they're flat on the floor, rest for a few seconds, then repeat the toe lift.

Next, lift your heels off the floor while your toes stay planted. Hold for 5 seconds, then relax for a few seconds.

Let your sheets breathe. Mom may have been a stickler about tucking in your bedsheets tightly, but loose sheets are actually healthier for your toes and legs, say doctors. Sleeping on your back under tightly tucked sheets can leave your toes flexed toward the tops of your feet, says Dr. Hamner. You may get cramps in the arches of your feet while sleeping in this position, he says. So pull the top sheet out from under the mattress and give yourself some slack before you go to sleep.

Charley Horses

A charley horse is a painful contraction in the thigh muscle. It can last a few seconds or a few minutes and is usually associated with athletic activity, says Dr. Hamner. Here's help for getting through one.

Try a thigh tamer. To treat a muscle cramp in the hamstring (back of the thigh), Dr. Hamner recommends that you try this stretch.

- Lie flat on your back on the floor.
- If the cramp is in your right leg, raise your leg by placing both hands just above or below the back of your knee and pulling it up, keeping it as straight as possible. Your left leg should be extended straight out on the floor.
- Pull your leg toward your chest as far as you comfortably can.
- Hold your leg firmly with your hands for at least 20 seconds until the cramp relaxes.
- If necessary, relax for a few seconds, then repeat to work out the cramp.

Harness the hams. For another hamstring stretch to fight a charley horse, Dr. Hamner suggests this exercise.

- Stand straight and clasp your hands behind your back.
- Keeping your head up and your knees and back as straight as possible, bend forward until you feel tightness in your hamstrings, but not pain.
- Hold this stretch for 20 seconds.
- Relax and try four more stretches.

Quell those quad cramps. Dr. Hamner recommends this stretch for cramps in the front of your thigh (the quadriceps muscle).

- Stand sideways next to or facing a wall and place your left hand against it for support.
- Bend your knee, grab your right foot with your right hand, and raise it behind your back, with your knee pointing down.
- Pull your leg back about 6 inches and tighten your buttocks, then pull back another 2 to 3 inches.
- Hold the stretch for 20 seconds.

Some Anti-Cramp Exercises

Here are a few exercises to head off cramps before they have you moaning in pain.

Pedal off the pain. A good cramp fighter is that trusty stationary bicycle that you keep in your bedroom or recreation room, says Dr. Levy.

Five to 10 minutes of steady pedaling at the lowest resistance setting may improve the circulation to the calf area and untie that muscle knot. Adding a regular cycling routine—even 15 minutes' worth—to your day may also help keep away future cramps, advises Dr. Levy.

Soak first. Treat yourself to a 10-minute relaxing soak in a warm tub before heading for bed. It will soothe your mind and calm your calves as well, says Dr. Hamner. As added insurance, try doing foot circles in the tub. While you're still seated in a comfortable position, pivot your ankles. Do 10 circles clockwise and then 10 counterclockwise with each foot. The warm water will increase bloodflow and help the muscles relax, he explains.

Neck Pain

Imagine trying to balance a 15-pound bowling bowl on your fingertips all day long. That's essentially what the seven bones and dozens of ligaments, muscles, and nerves in the neck have to do to properly perch and pivot your head.

When our neck bones, shock-absorbing disks, and muscles are flexible and strong, the head generally moves painlessly in all directions. But necks are under a lot of pressure. They're often undermined by tension, muscle spasms, arthritis, loss of bone mass, and even poor posture.

For immediate pain relief, apply heat or cold, says Mary Ann Keenan, M.D., director of neuro-orthopedics at Albert Einstein Medical Center in Philadelphia. You can apply a hot-water bottle or an ice pack to relieve your neck pain, she says. "They both work the same way, by increasing circulation to the area."

Low-sweat exercises can help ease—and prevent—many types of chronic neckaches, say doctors. Experts suggest two types of exercise that you might want to try: stretching exercises to improve the range of motion in your neck and strengthening exercises to help your muscles hold your head up proudly.

A word of caution: Your neck can be delicate. Doctors say that you should stop exercising immediately and see your physician if you experience numbness or sharp, intensifying pain during or after exercise.

Stretching for Full Mobility

A healthy neck is flexible enough to bend and twist easily in six directions: forward, backward, left, right, down toward the left shoulder, and down toward the right, says Kim Fagan, M.D., a sports medicine physician at the Alabama Sports Medicine and Orthopedic Center in Birmingham. Here are some easy stretching exercises that will give you good range of neck motion and relieve tension-induced pain. They can be done either sitting or standing. Dr. Fagan recommends moving in slow, controlled motions to get the most out of these stretches. She cautions not to stretch to the point of pain.

Head up and down. Start with your head erect, facing an imaginary spot on the wall at eye level. Slowly tilt your head forward until your chin touches your chest, as if you were about to nod off during a boring movie. Hold that stretch for 5 to 10 seconds. Then slowly tilt your head backward as far as you comfortably can without feeling pain. Hold that tilt for 5 to 10 seconds. Think of this action as a slow-motion nod of approval, says Dr. Fagan.

Do these head tilts twice a day, in the morning and evening. Start with 5 tilts, and gradually build up to 15 per session.

Try the slow no-no. Start with your head facing forward, then slowly rotate it to the left as far as you can. Hold that pose for 5 to 10 seconds. Relax, then slowly turn your head to the right as far as you can. Hold for 5 to 10 seconds, then relax. Start with 5 rotations, and gradually build up to 15 twice a day. As your neck muscles warm up, you should be able to turn farther to the left and right, says Dr. Fagan. This stretch not only helps relieve neck pain but also improves flexibility, making it easier to do things such as looking over your shoulder when you're backing out of the driveway.

Be a head rocker. Facing front, slowly tilt your head to the left, bringing your left ear toward your left shoulder. You should feel a warm stretch in your right neck muscles. Hold that stretch for 5 to 10 seconds, then relax and slowly tilt your head back to the right, bringing your right

Say No-No to Neck Pain

The first step in avoiding neck pain is proper posture. You have to avoid that head-forward hunch you favor when facing your computer or when scrunched up behind the steering wheel.

Holding your head forward often strains muscles and triggers spasms in the neck, says Robert Markison, M.D., a hand surgeon and associate clinical professor of surgery at the University of California, San Francisco. "When we put ourselves in a head-forward, limb-forward posture, we transmit up to three times the usual force through the neck, the spine, and the muscles around it," he says. To avoid neck pain, it's important to hold your head back, directly over your shoulders.

How's your posture? Check your alignment: Keep your spine as straight as you comfortably can while keeping your muscles relaxed. Your shoulders should be back, and your head and neck should be upright and directly over your shoulders, not tipped forward in front of your body.

ear toward your right shoulder. Hold for 5 to 10 seconds. Start with 5 of these complete head tilts and build up to 15 twice a day, recommends Dr. Fagan.

"You will actually feel a stretch, and as the muscles warm up, you should be able to get a better stretch with each one," says Dr. Fagan. "These stretches can help you deal with muscle pain and spasms." This stretch also helps relieve pain that comes from cradling a phone too long, she adds.

Face the clock. If you make time for neck stretches, activities such as working at a computer or reading a book should be less painful, says Thomas Meade, M.D., orthopedic surgeon and medical director of the Allentown Sports Medicine and Human Performance Center in Pennsylvania. Here's a stretch that he says should help.

Lie on your back with your knees bent and your feet flat on the floor. Imagine that you're looking upward into the face of a large clock. Using your nose as a pointer, try to move your head as if you were following the hour hand, clockwise from 1 o'clock to 12 o'clock. Then move your head counterclockwise with the same motion. Try five slow head circles in each direction. You can also try this standing up.

Neck-Strengthening Exercises

Once you have your neck muscles stretched, it's time to help make them stronger by building them up a bit. The stronger your neck muscles are, the less neck pain you'll feel. "Strengthening exercises can help prevent recurrence of muscle spasms and chronic pain in many cases," says Dr. Fagan. She recommends three "heads-up" exercises for strong, healthy neck muscles.

Rise up. To do this neck toner, lie on your back with your knees bent and your feet flat on the floor. Place a pillow under your head. While keeping your shoulders on the floor, tuck your chin and slowly lift your head toward your chest. Hold that position for 5 to 10 seconds and then lower your head. Try 5 of these at first, and gradually increase to 15 twice a day.

Head sideways. Lie on your right side on the floor with your legs straight and your head on a pillow. Lift your head up slowly toward your left shoulder as if you were peacefully waking up from a sound sleep. Hold the lift for 5 to 10 seconds and then gently lower your head back to the pillow. Repeat four more times, then lie on your left side and do five more head lifts. Move slowly for optimal muscle-toning effect, says Dr. Fagan.

Look skyward. The next time you lie on your stomach to read a novel or watch television, take a break and try this 1-minute neck muscle builder, says Dr. Fagan.

Lie facedown on a pillow with both hands on top of the pillow and your elbows pointed out. Lift your head straight up, tipping it backward and looking at the ceiling. Use your neck muscles, not your arms. Hold each lift for 5 to 10 seconds. With each successive lift, try to focus on a spot on the ceiling that requires greater range of motion backward. Do 5 lifts at first, and work up to 15 twice a day.

Osteoarthritis

Just like age, osteoarthritis can creep up on you. It starts out quietly, with some occasional stiffness. Later you may begin to feel some occasional joint pain. Human nature tells you to ignore it, but maybe you shouldn't. If you try some alternative therapies, you may be able to slow the disease before it does too much damage.

What's going on is ordinary wear and tear, for the most part. Take a look at the tread on a set of tires after you've racked up about 50,000 miles. The tires are worn, their surfaces uneven. The steel belts may even be peeking through in places.

Inside your body, it's the smooth, rubbery cushioning called cartilage that starts to erode. The gliding surface that normally acts as a shock absorber between your bones can become compressed and irregular. As the underlying cartilage and bone disintegrate, painful bone spurs can form in the joint. Ordinary movements can produce a grinding symphony of creaks and crackles.

While no one really knows what makes cartilage break down, heavy use of the joint seems to be a contributing factor. That's why osteoarthritis typically strikes the fingers, back, hips, or knees. Moreover, a joint injured in the past tends to develop arthritis sooner than one that's led a relatively pampered existence.

Scientists suspect that the damage from osteoarthritis may be due to an imbalance of enzymes in the joints. The right balance of enzymes allows for the natural breakdown and regeneration of cartilage. Too many enzymes, however, can cause the joint cartilage to break down faster than it can be rebuilt.

The Basics of Care

Signs of osteoarthritis show up in x-rays among most people over age 60. But only about a third have any of the typical symptoms of pain, stiffness, limited range of motion, or inflammation. That's one of the puzzling things about osteoarthritis. There doesn't seem to be a relationship between the amount of pain and the degree of joint damage. Some people never have more than a mild ache. Others develop crippling pain.

Still, arthritis is the leading cause of disability among Americans over age 15. Osteoarthritis, the most common form, affects 20.7 million people. While there aren't any miracle cures, there's a lot you can do to minimize the damage.

Maintain a healthy weight. People with osteoarthritis are more likely to be overweight. Research shows that losing weight can significantly reduce the risk of developing it. In a large study done in Framingham, Massachusetts, women who lost an average of 11 pounds were much less likely to get arthritis of the knee over the next 10 years than women who didn't shed the pounds.

Exercise. Low-impact activities like brisk walking, swimming, and biking are best at strengthening muscles and are easy on your joints. Stronger muscles help protect the joints by providing support and added stability.

Exercise also helps the joints absorb fluid and needed nutrients. Unlike muscle or bone, cartilage doesn't get its nutrients from blood. It soaks them up like a sponge from the fluid surrounding the joint. The more you exercise, the more you force fluid in and out of the joint.

Be careful with drugs. Aspirin and other similar drugs, called nonsteroidal anti-inflammatory drugs (NSAIDs), focus on reducing arthritis pain, but that pain relief isn't in your long-term interest, according to doctors. While NSAIDs are easing the pain, they can actually speed up joint deterioration. Natural measures attempt to slow the progression of the disease and preserve cartilage and bone by providing the proper nutrients in the right amounts.

Ensure a steady supply of building materials. One arthritis treatment that has hit the spotlight is the supplement combo glucosamine and chondroitin, two substances that your body makes to help build and protect cartilage. When taken together, glucosamine and chondroitin seem to slow the loss of cartilage from the joint by pumping more cartilage-generating nutrients into the body, says Amal Das, M.D., an orthopedic surgeon with Hendersonville Orthopedic Associates in North Carolina.

Scientists believe that glucosamine somehow stimulates the cartilage cells to produce two important compounds that are the building blocks of cartilage. Once you have taken it for 8 weeks, the supplement seems to provide pain relief comparable to that of ibuprofen, but without side effects.

While the research seems to paint a clear picture of the role of glucosamine supplements, the image is still fuzzy when it comes to chondroitin, says Lauri Aesoph, N.D., a health-care consultant in Sioux Falls, South Dakota, and author of *How to Eat Away Arthritis*. Glucosamine is a small molecule that is readily absorbed. Chondroitin is huge by comparison. Ranging from 50 to 300 times larger, it is unable to pass through the intestinal wall intact. But apparently, the two supplements seem to work best together, says Dr. Das. "Chondroitin inhibits the enzyme that breaks down cartilage. We're really excited about it because it may be the first disease-modifying agent for arthritis. It's the first medicine to give us hope."

Because the pair works best by preserving the cartilage you have left, don't wait until you're in agonizing pain to start on a supplement program, advises Dr. Das. If you've been diagnosed with arthritis, get your doctor's approval first, then take 500 milligrams of glucosamine and 400 milligrams of chondroitin sulfate twice a day, says Dr. Das. From the time you start the double dose, allow from 2 weeks to 4 months to let the supplements do their work. You can continue to take them indefinitely.

Although the patients in Dr. Das's study took glucosamine hydrochloride, many naturopathic physicians typically recommend taking glucosamine sulfate because it is the type that has been tested most thoroughly in clinical trials.

You might see on store shelves a third form of glucosamine, called N-acetylglucosamine, commonly referred to as NAG. While the label may state that NAG is better utilized and therefore more effective than glucosamine sulfate, no research has yet been conducted that would prove or disprove that claim, says Dr. Aesoph.

Apply antioxidant relief. Antioxidants—especially vitamin C, vitamin E, and beta-carotene—are another means of preventing your cartilage from wearing away.

"Arthritis is known to increase free radical production, so your need for antioxidant nutrients increases," says Dr. Aesoph. Those free radicals are free-roaming, unstable molecules that can set off a chain reaction in the body, aging cells prematurely and sometimes harming the genetic material. Research has shown that diets high in antioxidants help reduce pain and cartilage deterioration.

To protect your cartilage and quell aches and pains, take 1,000 milligrams of buffered vitamin C three times a day, says Ruth Bar-Shalom, a naturopathic doctor in Fairbanks, Alaska.

Studies show that vitamin E offers relief from inflammation. To get benefits, include 600 IU of vitamin E and 10,000 IU of beta-carotene in your daily antioxidant regimen, says Dr. Bar-Shalom.

Get crucial cartilage nutrients. If you're not getting the right nutrients, your body cannot make and maintain cartilage. In addition to antioxidants, four key players in the production process are pantothenic acid, zinc, copper, and vitamin D. A deficiency of any one of these can cause accelerated joint degeneration, says Dr. Bar-Shalom.

Although many mainstream doctors view osteoarthritis as an inevitable part of growing older, naturopathic doctors contend that it is a metabolic disorder brought on by the body's inability to regenerate bone and cartilage. Taking a holistic approach to treating arthritis, a naturopathic doctor looks at imbalances that may be occurring in the whole body, then attempts to correct those imbalances.

Dr. Bar-Shalom customizes the diet plan for each of her patients, but in general she suggests starting with a low-fat diet that is high in fiber and complex carbohydrates and drinking at least eight 8-ounce glasses of water a day. Then you'll be ready to supplement a healthy diet with other crucial cartilage nutrients.

Pantothenic acid is one of those nutrients, according to Dr. Bar-Shalom. Without pantothenic acid, cartilage can't grow. Studies have found that supplements of this B vitamin relieved arthritis symptoms, and research with animals has shown that if animals have a profound deficiency of pantothenic acid, their cartilage will stop growing.

Pantothenic acid is found in foods such as whole grains, legumes, fish, and poultry. The Daily Value is 10 milligrams, but Dr. Bar-Shalom recommends 12.5 milligrams of pantothenic acid plus 50 milligrams of vitamin B_6 daily to encourage your body's ability to regenerate cartilage as it's being lost.

Add zinc and D. Zinc is another of the body's much-needed resources. While virtually all cells contain zinc, some of the highest concentrations are in bone. If you have a deficiency, your body's ability to make collagen—the "glue" for your connective tissues—is seriously impaired.

To promote tissue repair, Dr. Bar-Shalom recommends a daily dose of 45 milligrams of zinc. Doses above 20 milligrams must be taken under medical supervision. When zinc intake is high, it can interfere with your absorption of copper, so Dr. Bar-Shalom adds 1 milligram of copper to the daily supplement regimen.

Underneath degenerating cartilage, bone also deteriorates. Vitamin D, a necessary nutrient for absorption of calcium, can help preserve bone and slow the loss of cartilage, says Dr. Aesoph. You can get vitamin D from exposure to sunlight or from fortified milk. If you're over 50 or have osteoarthritis, you should supplement with 400 IU of vitamin D daily.

Turn off inflammation. The word *arthritis*, derived from Greek, means "inflammation of the joint." While this definition certainly applies to another kind of arthritis—rheumatoid arthritis—the term is somewhat contradictory in referring to osteoarthritis. People with osteoarthritis generally have very little inflammation.

Nevertheless, doctors do recommend anti-inflammatory medicines such as aspirin and ibuprofen for pain relief. Are they effective?

While they do relieve pain, these over-the-counter drugs, along with many prescription-strength pain relievers, take a toll on your body, says Dr. Aesoph. Their long-term use has been associated with ulcers and gastrointestinal bleeding.

"The side effect that is often overlooked is that they prevent cartilage repair," says Jody Noé, N.D., a naturopathic doctor at the Brattleboro Naturopathic Clinic in Vermont. Those pain relievers interfere with the way the body creates new tissue around the joints, she notes. They actually accelerate the destruction of cartilage.

Given those side effects, it certainly makes sense to look for an alternative way to stop pain and inflammation. For drug-free relief, take 1 tablespoon of flaxseed oil and 500 milligrams of black currant oil (or three capsules of evening primrose oil) every day, says David Perlmutter, M.D., a neurologist in Naples, Florida, and author of *Lifeguide*. Studies show that these two supplements switch on your body's natural inflammation-fighting powers.

Go for gentle pain relief. Supplementing with the herb devil's claw can sometimes relieve joint pain, says Dr. Bar-Shalom. Studies have shown that this herb provides some relief from pain and inflammation. The active substance at work is harpagoside, a compound found in the tuberous roots of the plant. It reduces inflammation in the joints and helps stimulate cortisol, your body's natural version of pain-relieving cortisone. A sensible dose to start with is 400 milligrams of dry standardized extract three times a day, says Dr. Noé. Do not use devil's claw, however, if you have gastric or duodenal ulcers.

Although better known for its power to defuse migraines, feverfew also inhibits an enzyme that causes inflammation, says Betzy Bancroft, a professional member of the American Herbalists Guild in Washington, New Jersey.

To control joint pain, take 125 milligrams of standardized extract containing at least 0.2 percent parthenolide or 1 to 3 milliliters of tincture daily, says Dr. Noé.

Say yes to yucca. Yucca, an herb with more than 40 species, is recommended for relief of joint pain, says Jill Stansbury, N.D., assistant professor of botanical medicine and chair of the botanical medicine department at the National College of Naturopathic Medicine in Portland, Oregon.

In treating arthritis, herbalists believe that yucca works best when it is used with other herbs that fight inflammation, such as ginger, turmeric, devil's claw, angelica, and willow bark.

One theory is that the plant eases arthritis pain by reducing the absorption of wastes produced by bacteria in the intestine. "We think that arthritis might have its roots in the digestive process," says Dr. Stansbury.

A link between the gut and sore joints may sound farfetched, but an animal study has shown that an accumulation of bacterial wastes in the intestine can impair cartilage growth. When your food is not broken down properly during digestion, undesirable bacteria can multiply rapidly and produce toxic substances called endotoxins. If absorbed through the walls of the intestine, these toxins can travel through your body and inflame the connective tissue, says Dr. Stansbury.

Naturopathic physicians believe that yucca may decrease absorption of endotoxins in the intestine. It works gradually, however, and sometimes takes up to 3 months before providing signs of improvement, says Dr. Stansbury.

Yucca may be difficult to find in your local health food store. You're more likely to find it as part of an herbal arthritis formula. Dosage recommendations on the package tend to be on the low side, says Dr. Stansbury. If the formula gives a dosage range such as ½ to 1 teaspoon of liquid two to five times a day or one or two capsules two to four times a day, she recommends aiming for the high end.

Try niacinamide—with caution. Since the 1940s, some doctors have recommended niacinamide, a form of niacin, to treat osteoarthritis. There is growing evidence that large doses of this B-complex vitamin can improve joint flexibility and reduce inflammation.

The niacinamide form of the vitamin is used because it produces fewer side effects, such as the uncomfortable flushing and rash associated with niacin. How it works is still uncertain. Doctors and researchers think that large amounts of extra niacinamide somehow improve the ability of the cartilage to repair itself.

Before you stock up on this supplement, check with your doctor. The 3,000-milligram daily dose successfully used in one study is 150 times the Daily Value of 20 milligrams. "At high doses there is a significant risk for liver damage," says Dr. Noé. "You need to be monitored by a health-care professional when you're taking high-range doses."

Anyone taking more than 1,500 milligrams of niacinamide a day should have a blood test for liver enzymes after 3 months of treatment, Dr. Noé advises. If the levels are elevated, the dosage will have to be reduced. Nausea is an early-warning sign of stress on the liver.

Rheumatoid Arthritis

If you have rheumatoid arthritis, your body's infection-fighting immune cells decide that *you're* the enemy. They attack your joints and cause inflammation, with pain, redness, heat, swelling, and tissue damage. The inflammation doesn't always confine itself to joints, either, says Andrew Rubman, N.D., director of the Southbury Clinic for Traditional Medicine in Connecticut and consultant to the Office of Complementary and Alternative Medicine at the National Institutes of Health. "Other organs, such as the skin, heart, and lungs, can be affected," he says.

Although arthritis is potentially crippling, there are things you can do that may help control it. Here's what doctors recommend.

Reach for the "right" pain reliever. Not all pain relievers are the same—at least for people with arthritis. "People with inflammatory arthritis should get more relief from aspirin or ibuprofen (Advil) but may get more stomach irritation with these," says Paul Caldron, D.O., a clinical rheumatologist and researcher at the Arthritis Center in Phoenix. For over-the-counter pain relief without stomach irritation, he recommends acetaminophen (Tylenol). Recommended doses of these drugs should not be exceeded, nor should you continue regular dosing for more than 3 weeks without consulting your physician.

Get hot on hot-pepper cream. Research shows you can ease the pain by rubbing the joint with an over-the-counter ointment called Zostrix, made from capsaicin—the stuff that puts the hot in hot peppers. "You need to apply it three or four times a day on the affected area for at least 2 weeks before you'll see any improvement. An initial burning sensation at the site is not unusual for the first few days, but this goes away with continued application," says Esther Lipstein Kresch, M.D., an assistant professor of medicine at the Albert Einstein College of Medicine of Yeshiva University in New York City who has studied the effectiveness of capsaicin cream. "I also advise washing your hands immediately after you apply it—or even wearing gloves when you apply it—because it can sting, and you don't want to get it in your eyes." (Sorry, but eating hot peppers won't help relieve arthritis.)

Learn your food "triggers." "Some people with rheumatoid arthritis seem to flare up after eating certain foods—especially alcohol, milk, tomatoes, and certain nuts," says Dr. Caldron. "Although there's really no telling what your trigger might be, if you notice that your condition worsens after eating a certain food, then listen to your body and avoid that food."

Use ice and heat judiciously. Although both ice packs and heat packs can provide some relief, don't use either for more than 10 minutes at a time, advises Dr. Caldron. Ice usually is used to prevent swelling but may also douse pain; heat in small doses may promote muscle relaxation and soothe pain.

Use a dehumidifier. Keeping the humidity in your house constant can help calm arthritis pain caused by weather changes, says Joseph Hollander, M.D., professor emeritus of medicine at the University of Pennsylvania Hospital in Philadelphia. When rain is on the way, the sudden increase in humidity and decrease in air pressure can affect bloodflow to arthritic joints, which become increasingly stiff until the storm actually starts. If you close the windows and turn on a dehumidifier—or run the air conditioner in summer—you may be able to eliminate this short-term but significant pain.

Natural Alternatives

Alternative practitioners attack rheumatoid arthritis on several additional fronts, says Jody Noé, N.D., a naturopathic doctor at the Brattleboro Naturopathic Clinic in Vermont. They use anti-inflammatory nutrients and herbs. Often these supplements are prescribed in large doses, so you'll need the advice of a practitioner or a doctor before you start taking them.

Some of the recommended supplements also work to restore proper immunity and to get the adrenal glands functioning better. These glands, located above the kidneys, are powerful little organs that secrete hormones, such as epinephrine and steroids, that affect many organ functions and influence the use of energy throughout your body.

Alternative practitioners also try to address what they believe are potential triggers of autoimmune diseases such as rheumatoid arthritis. Naturopathic doctors believe that one trigger is increased intestinal permeability, or "leaky gut," a condition that occurs when molecules of incompletely digested food or bacterial fragments appear to seep through the walls of the intestine, setting off an immune response.

People also have allergic reactions to foods, and if you see an alternative practitioner about rheumatoid arthritis, you're likely to be questioned closely about what foods you eat and when. Realizing that adrenal gland problems can arise from too much physical or emotional stress, alternative practitioners may try to treat the stress as a way of avoiding an autoimmune reaction. If you've been diagnosed with rheumatoid arthritis and want to try these options, get your doctor's approval first.

Ax inflammation with antioxidants. Any time you have inflammation, there's production of free radicals, unstable molecules that can harm surrounding cells, causing what's called oxidative damage. Some nutrients that may help stop free radicals and prevent that damage include vitamins E and C, beta-carotene, selenium, and zinc.

Several studies have shown that the risk of rheumatoid arthritis is highest among people with the lowest blood levels of these nutrients. Other studies suggest that whether or not people are deficient, these nutrients may help reduce the arthritis symptoms.

In a Belgian study, 15 women with rheumatoid arthritis who took 160 micrograms of selenium or 200 micrograms of selenium-enriched yeast every day for 4 months experienced significant improvement in joint movement and strength. Another study showed that people with rheumatoid arthritis who took 600 international units (IU) of vitamin E twice a day had a significant reduction in pain compared with people who took pills with no vitamin E (placebos).

Researchers at the University of Washington in Seattle found that people with rheumatoid arthritis who took 50 milligrams of zinc three times a day for 3 months experienced significant improvement in joint swelling and morning stiffness with the aid of the supplements. With the zinc, it also took them less time to walk certain distances than when they were not taking it.

"Zinc helps your body make an important inflammation-fighting enzyme called superoxide dismutase," says Dr. Noé. She cautions, however, that this doesn't mean that you should take the amounts of zinc that were used in the study; those amounts of zinc should not be taken without medical supervision.

Dr. Noé recommends a daily mixture of antioxidant nutrients, including 1,000 to 3,000 milligrams of vitamin C in divided doses, 400 to 1,000 IU of vitamin E, 200 to 400 micrograms of selenium, and 15 to 30 milligrams of zinc picolinate or citrate.

You can also take 1 to 2 milligrams a day of copper and 5 to 15 milligrams of manganese, suggests Dr. Noé. Both of these trace minerals help the body make its own antioxidants. Be careful not to take higher doses of these two, however, as they can be toxic in large amounts.

"A good multivitamin/mineral will cover a lot of these nutritional bases," Dr. Noé says. To maximize absorption from a multi, she suggests taking capsules with meals.

Turn to friendly fats. You might reduce the amount of inflammation-generating chemicals that your body produces by changing the kinds of fats you eat, Dr. Noé says. "Meat and other animal foods provide your body with something called arachidonic acid, which is used to make pro-inflammatory biochemicals," she explains.

There are other fats that don't have the effect of stimulating inflammation. Certain plant oils, as well as oils from cold-water fish such as mackerel, follow a chemical pathway that is pretty much neutral, according to Dr. Noé. Thus, if those are your primary sources of fat, you'll be a lot less likely to aggravate arthritis symptoms.

At least six studies have shown that diets rich in fish oil, which contains omega-3 fatty acids, help reduce the pain and stiffness of rheumatoid arthritis as well as the biochemical signs of inflammation. Evidence so far suggests that taking 3,000 to 6,000 milligrams a day of these fatty acids seems to have an anti-inflammatory effect, Dr. Noé says. Good food sources are herring, salmon, tuna, sardines, mackerel, and anchovies.

Two studies also suggest that gamma-linolenic acid (GLA), a kind of fatty acid found in certain plant oils, may reduce the symptoms of rheumatoid arthritis. In one study, people took 2.8 grams a day of GLA for 1 year. At the end of that time, 76 percent showed improvement.

Dr. Noé recommends taking 1,000 to 1,500 milligrams a day of eicosapentaenoic acid (EPA) and 500 to 700 milligrams a day of docosahexaenoic acid (DHA), both of which are active ingredients in fish-oil supplements. She also suggests supplementing with 500 to 1,000 milligrams of GLA from evening primrose, borage, or black currant oil.

Improve digestion. Some kinds of arthritis have a clear link with inflammatory bowel disease. Two with confirmed links are arthritis of the knees, ankles, and wrists and ankylosing spondylitis (rheumatoid arthritis of the spine).

These links, as well as other clues, have suggested to doctors of alternative medicine that digestive problems can play a role in rheumatoid arthritis. Here's where the leaky gut theory comes in. If incompletely digested food and bacterial fragments are seeping through the intestinal lining into the bloodstream, so the thinking goes, maybe they're setting off an improper immune response that ends up causing rheumatoid arthritis.

"It's possible to do tests that can confirm if someone is having an immune reaction that could cause rheumatoid arthritis," Dr. Noé says. Your rheumatologist or a naturopathic doctor can order these tests.

In addition, she recommends nutritional supplements that nourish and rebuild the intestinal lining and restore good bacteria to the bowel. Some foods that commonly aggravate leaky gut are wheat gluten, corn, and dairy products.

"I may also recommend enzymes that help break down food for proper digestion if tests suggest that someone's pancreas is not producing enough for normal digestion," Dr. Noé says.

To provide nourishment directly to intestinal cells, she suggests a large number of supplements that are specifically used to treat autoimmune diseases like rheumatoid arthritis and lupus. They include:

- 500 to 750 milligrams of the amino acid glutamine.
- 100 to 300 milligrams of gamma-oryzanol, a component of rice bran oil.
- 50 to 100 milligrams of fructooligosaccharides (FOS), taken two or three times a day between meals. (Fructooligosaccharides are naturally occurring sugars that help to promote the growth of friendly bacteria in the intestines.)
- One or two capsules two or three times a day of a supplement containing various forms of lactobacillus and other so-called friendly bacteria—*Lactobacillus acidophilus*, *L. rhamnosus*, *L. casei*, *L. plantarum*, *Bifidobacterium bifidum*, *B. longum*, and *B. breve*. The recommended dose has 2 to 5 billion active organisms per capsule.
- 500 to 1,000 milligrams of 10X U.S.P. of digestive enzymes. (10X U.S.P. is a measure of strength, listed on the bottle.)
- A mixture of other enzymes derived from plants, including 12,500 to 18,000 U.S.P. of protease, 2,675 U.S.P. of lipase, 12,000 to 27,000 U.S.P. of amylase, and 175 CU(2) of cellulase.

Dr. Noé says that these supplements are safe to take on a continuous basis as long as you get your doctor's approval and remain under supervision. Some of the supplements may be available only through a naturopathic physician or a holistic doctor.

Ease aches the spicy way. Turmeric, an Indian spice, contains an anti-inflammatory and antioxidant compound called curcumin that might be helpful for people with rheumatoid arthritis, especially during flare-ups, says Dr. Rubman. "In animals, curcumin has excellent anti-inflammatory and antioxidant effects, without any toxicity," he says.

When curcumin is present, the body is much less likely to form the compounds that are instrumental in causing inflammation, according to Dr. Rubman. Research with humans is still sketchy, but some preliminary studies have suggested benefits.

The recommended dose of curcumin is 400 to 600 milligrams three times a day with or without food, Dr. Rubman says. If you don't notice some relief within 10 days, stop taking it. It is safe to take indefinitely as long as you don't have a digestive problem, but for best results, he recommends seeking the care of a naturopathic physician. Curcumin is available from naturopathic doctors and is sold at health food stores.

Bring in bromelain. To enhance absorption of curcumin and add more anti-inflammatory power, supplement manufacturers sometimes mix curcumin with bromelain, an enzyme found in pineapple, Dr. Rubman says.

"Bromelain can activate compounds that break down fibrin, tissue that blocks off areas of inflammation," Dr. Rubman explains. He points out that the fibrin blocks blood vessels, which can prevent tissues from draining and cause them to swell.

Bromelain also blocks the production of compounds produced during inflammation that increase swelling and cause pain.

The usual dosage for bromelain, according to Dr. Rubman, is 400 to 600 milligrams three times a day, taken on an empty stomach at the same time as curcumin. Mixtures of bromelain and curcumin in a ratio designed to reduce inflammation are available at some health food stores or from a naturopathic doctor.

Get going with ginger. Ginger, the spice used in baking and a relative of curcumin, has anti-inflammatory and antioxidant properties that make it helpful for rheumatoid arthritis, Dr. Rubman says. In two small studies, ginger helped to reduce muscle stiffness, pain, and swelling.

You can take ginger instead of curcumin if you prefer, he says. The doses he recommends are 100 to 200 milligrams three times a day of ginger extract standardized to contain 20 percent gingerol and shogaol, the active ingredients. You also have the option of 8 to 10 grams (about 1½ tablespoons) of fresh ginger or 2 to 4 grams (about 1 teaspoon) of dry powdered ginger daily. Do not use the dried root or powder if you have gallstones.

Ginger can be especially soothing if your rheumatoid arthritis includes gastrointestinal problems. If you tend to "run hot," as Dr. Rubman puts it—if you tend to sweat a lot or have hot, swollen joints—you're better off avoiding ginger, he says.

Sciatica

If all your nerves were a network of roads, the sciatic nerve would be a busy interstate highway. All of the nerve impulses transmitted to and from the lower half of your body must pass through the sciatic nerve, the largest and longest in the body. From its roots in the spinal cord, the thick conduit branches through the buttocks and down the back of each leg to the foot. Pain that follows this route is called sciatica.

Pressure on the nerve in the spinal area is normally the cause of sciatica. The sensation can vary from mild tingling in your foot to searing pains that shoot down your leg.

Sciatica often begins after you've done some customary movement that never caused pain previously. Smokers, people who do a lot of heavy lifting, and people with osteoporosis or arthritis are at highest risk for developing sciatica.

To discover what's causing your pain, you'd have to look closely at an x-ray of your spinal column, particularly the disks, circular sections of cartilage that are assigned the job of cushioning the bones and sheltering the nerve that runs alongside your spine. If you're under age 40 and you get sciatica, it's likely that one of those disks has slipped and is bulging between the vertebrae in your spine. Since the nerve runs alongside the spine, the off-kilter disk puts pressure on it.

If you're hit with sciatica when you're over 40, the cause is also disk-related, but in a somewhat different way. At that age your disks are starting to become dehydrated. The shrinking disks can cause the spine to compress, increasing pressure on the nerve.

Do you get the pain most when you cough or sneeze? That's just one sign that your sciatic nerve is probably pinched. You really can't diagnose yourself from that clue alone, however, so you should see a doctor to be sure of the origin of the pain, says Barbara Silbert, D.C., N.D., a chiropractor and naturopathic doctor in Newburyport, Massachusetts. Lower-back pain and intermittent claudication—pain in the legs caused by poor arterial bloodflow—are often mistaken for sciatic pain, notes Dr. Silbert.

Feel Better Fast

Any time you have back pain for more than 2 to 3 days, you should see your doctor to rule out serious illness or injury, suggests Sheila Reid, therapy coordinator at the Spine Institute of New England in Williston, Vermont. But once your doctor rules out other things and positively identifies sciatica, here are some ways to find relief and help prevent future attacks.

Apply ice. To help reduce pain and swelling, apply ice where you feel sciatica pain, Reid says. To protect your skin, place a towel between your back and the ice pack. Ice may be used for 15 to 20 minutes every hour. Or switch to the warmth of a heating pad, shower, or bath, she says. Heat relaxes muscles.

Reach over the counter. Nonprescription pain relievers such as acetaminophen (Tylenol), ibuprofen (Advil), or naproxen (Aleve) may help relieve temporary discomfort, says Steven Mandel, M.D., clinical professor of neurology at Thomas Jefferson University Hospital in Philadelphia. But be sure to ask your physician first. Even over-the-counter medicines can have side effects.

Please sit up. Prolonged sitting may aggravate your discomfort because it reverses the normal curve in your back, says John E. Thomassy, D.C., chiropractor in private practice in Virginia Beach, Virginia. Sitting may compress disks and weaken lower-back ligaments and muscles. When you sit, maintain good posture. Don't slouch. Keep your knees level with your hips, your feet flat on the floor, and your back straight.

Get the angles right. If you are working at a desk or computer, adjust your chair so your elbows can be positioned at a 90-degree angle, with your forearms parallel to the floor, advises Dr. Thomassy. Tuck a small pillow behind your back to help you sit up straight and promote the normal curves in your spine.

Break things up. Take frequent breaks when you're working, Reid says. Get up and walk around every half-hour. If you're traveling in a car, avoid prolonged time behind the wheel or even in the passenger seat. Make frequent rest stops—at least every hour or so.

Helping Your Body Douse Inflammation

Because sciatica almost always involves a mechanical problem with your back, you may need massage or chiropractic adjustment. In severe cases surgery may be necessary to free the nerve. More often the doctor will simply prescribe some bed rest. You might also want to try some natural supplements that can help relieve inflammation and relax spastic muscles, says Dr. Silbert.

The key to drug-free relief is to turn on your body's natural inflammation-fighting powers, says David Perlmutter, M.D., a neurologist in Naples, Florida, and author of *Lifeguide*. Nutritional supplements can reprogram the chemical process that produces pain signals. Moreover, nutrients influence the complicated inflammation process.

"Obviously, the body must have its own ways of reducing inflammation," says Dr. Perlmutter. "The entire process of turning inflammation on and off is controlled by a group of hormonelike molecules called prostaglandins." According to Dr. Perlmutter, there are basically two groups of prostaglandins. One group is the starter kit, the bad ones, which initiate inflammation. The other is a "tone group," the good ones, which reduce the flare-up.

Here are supplements that inhibit the production of bad prostaglandins and promote the production of good prostaglandins.

Fight the flames. Bromelain, an enzyme found in pineapple, is the jack-of-all-trades when it comes to fighting inflammation. In a study of 146 boxers, researchers showed that bromelain significantly sped up the healing process when the boxers were injured.

Quercetin, just one of more than 800 bioflavonoids that have been identified, works best with bromelain to block the inflammation process. Naturopathic doctors believe that bromelain helps the body absorb the quercetin, so they often prescribe the two together, says Dr. Silbert. Quercetin is rich in powerful antioxidants that stop the damaging effects of free radicals, the unstable molecules that damage cells.

When the pain of sciatica strikes, take up to 1,000 milligrams of bromelain and 500 milligrams of quercetin four times a day between meals, says Dr. Silbert. The strength of a particular batch of bromelain is measured in milk clotting units (mcu) or gelatin-dissolving units (gdu). The higher the mcu number, the greater its strength. Look for a supplement with a strength between 1,800 and 2,400 mcu or 1,080 and 1,440 gdu.

Beware of bromelain supplements that merely list weight in milligrams; if the measurement isn't listed on the label, you can assume that you are getting a cheap, ineffective preparation, cautions Jacob Schor, N.D., a naturopathic doctor in Denver and president of the Colorado Association of Naturopathic Doctors.

Find help with fatty acids. Any type of inflammation responds well to the essential fatty acids found in fish oil, flaxseed oil, and evening primrose oil.

To reprogram your pain process, take 1 tablespoon of flaxseed oil and 500 milligrams of black currant oil (or three capsules of evening primrose oil) every day, says Dr. Perlmutter. These two supplements are rich in omega-3 and omega-6 essential fatty acids, which your body needs but cannot make. By adding them to your diet, you can stimulate your body to produce increased levels of good prostaglandins and reduce inflammation.

If you want to use fish oil instead of flaxseed oil, take 1,000 milligrams two to four times a day, says Priscilla Evans, N.D., a naturopathic doctor at the Community Wholistic Health Center in Chapel Hill, North Carolina.

Take time for turmeric. During intense flare-ups, add some turmeric. This yellow spice contains one of nature's most powerful anti-inflammatory drugs, a chemical called curcumin. The herb has been used for thousands of years in India's traditional Ayurvedic medicine to treat pain and inflammation.

Several clinical studies show that curcumin has an anti-inflammatory action. Don't reach into your spice cupboard for relief, however. Instead, opt for capsules of standardized extract that contain 97 percent pure curcumin.

When pain is acute, Dr. Evans advises people to take 250 to 500 milligrams three times a day. But you shouldn't take turmeric as a remedy if you are pregnant or have severe stomach acid, ulcers, gallstones, or a bile duct obstruction.

If you're taking natural supplements, you should start to see some improvement in about 2 weeks. Stick with the dosages to get the desired effect, says Dr. Evans.

"We lose sight of the fact that many nutritional and herbal supplements are more like foods than drugs. Dosages are important because taking just one capsule a day is not going to do much for your symptoms," she says. "In many cases you have to take a pretty large dose of fish oil or curcumin to get an effect."

Reach for the relaxation recipe. Sometimes pain and tingling can be due to muscle spasms in the piriformis muscle, a pear-shaped muscle in the buttocks that surrounds the sciatic nerve. Relaxing this muscle can help relieve pain, says Dr. Evans.

Naturopaths often use a mixture of soothing herbs such as valerian, passionflower, and kava kava to promote muscle relaxation. Although valerian has become a staple on drugstore shelves, where it is sold as a sleep aid, its powers of reprieve go beyond sleep.

"Valerian is also great for easing tension and for general pain relief," says Dr. Evans. It contains substances known as volatile oils that work together to make you sleepy and relax your muscles.

Sometimes your sciatic nerve is in the grip of a spastic muscle, and that no-win tug-of-war is at the root of the pain. Your doctor will need to confirm if a spastic muscle is the source of your pain. If it is, taking 150 milligrams of valerian three times a day may help, says Dr. Evans.

Shingles

If you had chicken pox in childhood, your parents probably told you that you'd never get it again. That's good news to any kid who has just endured the little blisters, the itching, and the fever that are all signs of chicken pox.

It's too bad that your parents were wrong.

The same virus that causes chicken pox—the varicella zoster virus—can continue to live an undercover existence in your nerve cells, and it may emerge later. The second time around, you don't get the childhood version of itchy, blotchy chicken pox. Instead, you get the adult version, shingles, which is characterized by searing pain and lesions that can leave good-size scars.

It's hard to tell why the virus re-emerges in some people and not others, and impossible to tell when it's going to crop up again. Certainly, elderly people get it more often than young people, and some individuals are more likely to develop shingles when they're under severe stress or when their immune systems have been weakened. Adults may get shingles after an illness. For cancer patients who are undergoing chemotherapy, compromised immune systems may be a factor in bringing on shingles.

What characterizes all of these situations is a weakened immune system in which your body's disease-fighting soldiers, the antibodies, are in short supply.

"The virus looks for the right opportunity, when your antibody production is down," says William Warnock, N.D., a naturopathic doctor in Shelburne, Vermont. "Stress is one of the biggest causes of reduced antibody production. When people become stressed, they don't eat right, they don't sleep well, and their immune systems just don't function as well."

Typically during a shingles outbreak, you have tingling and pain around your torso, neck, or face. Lesions, or small blisters, may break out on the skin near the site of the infected nerve. The pain often lasts from 2 to 4 weeks, but in some cases it can last for months. If it does, you've moved from shingles to a condition known as postherpetic neuralgia.

Fight the virus head-on. Once it gets loose, there's no cure for the varicella zoster virus, but there may be ways to slow it down or limit damage during the outbreak. Doctors frequently prescribe an antiviral drug such as acyclovir (Zovirax) or famciclovir (Famvir) to shorten the course of the infection. In order to hasten healing, treatment should be started within 2 to 3 days of the first appearance of the small blisters.

Pull the reins on pain. With your physician's okay, reach for acetaminophen (Tylenol) or another mild over-the-counter pain reliever such as ibuprofen (Advil), says Karl R. Beutner, M.D., Ph.D., associate clinical professor and researcher in the department of dermatology at the University of California, San Francisco.

Dry out the blisters. You can't do a lot to get rid of the shingles rash; it must run its course. But you can help dry the oozing blisters, says Dr. Beutner. Apply calamine lotion or use Burrow's solution made from Domeboro tablets, both available in drugstores. As the wet solutions evaporate from your skin, they also steal moisture from the blisters.

Turn to echinacea. You may be able to boost your immunity and help fight the virus with some herbs, says Dr. Warnock. They work best if you take them as soon as you know you have an outbreak of the virus. Although you can take an herbal tincture, he recommends taking one 300-milligram capsule of standardized extract three times a day.

If you use capsules of dried echinacea root, he recommends 2,000 milligrams three times a day. Since echinacea is also safe at higher doses, you can take even more than the specified dose if you find it effective. "I'd do a high dose for a short period—just a few days. That's when it's most effective," he says.

Aid healing with astragalus. While echinacea speeds white blood cells to the infection site, you can add astragalus to help with the healing process. This herb provides what is known as deep immune support, working within the bone marrow where immune cells are manufactured, says Anne McClenon, N.D., a naturopathic doctor at the Compass Family Health Center in Plymouth, Massachusetts. You can take astragalus in capsule form, following the directions on the label.

"Astragalus provides immune support on a long-term basis. That's important because people who get shingles may have a weakened immune system that needs to be built up again," she says. "I'd recommend taking it for 4 to 6 months."

Beat the pain with a B vitamin. Shingles is not just painful; it's *intensely* painful. Because your nerves carry the virus and the virus causes inflammation, having shingles is like having a raw wound inside your nervous system. Even a light touch can give you a jolt, while something as innocuous as a tight shirt can give you a full day of misery.

Vitamin B_{12} seems to maintain the fatty membranes that sheathe and insulate the nerves, says Dr. McClenon. There's also evidence that it reduces the inflammation of the nerve where the virus is causing pain, and it may even shorten the length of the illness.

Some people with shingles take vitamin B_{12} injections, says Dr. McClenon. If the idea of an injection doesn't appeal to you, you can get B_{12} tablets to place under your tongue (sublingual). Although some people have difficulty absorbing B_{12}, most people can absorb at least some of the vitamin this way.

"It definitely speeds healing," says Dr. McClenon, "and it may lessen the chance of a person's getting the postherpetic neuralgic pain." She suggests taking a 2,000-microgram dose of sublingual B_{12} each day during the course of the infection.

Limit the lesions with herbal treatments. The skin outbreaks and pain of shingles can sometimes be eased with herbal treatments that you can apply directly to the surface of the skin. Licorice root comes in a gel or ointment form that you rub directly on painful skin areas. It seems to interfere with the spread of the virus, says Dr. Warnock. Licorice gel (Licrogel) is available from your physician or chiropractor. You can also ask your health food store to order a brand called Licroderm.

Although naturopathic doctors find that St. John's wort oil applied to the unbroken skin acts as an anti-inflammatory, it also is used to relieve pain and strengthen nerves, says Dr. McClenon. "Thus, it's a good topical treatment for any kind of nerve pain. I would continue to use it for the residual pain that may linger after the outbreak."

Say "aloe-ahhh." The thin, milky liquid inside the leaves of the aloe vera plant may also help soothe the blisters, says Richard P. Huemer, M.D., holistic practitioner in Lancaster, California. If you have an aloe houseplant, cut a leaf and smooth the liquid over your skin. Or try an over-the-counter aloe lotion.

Fight fire with fire. Many over-the-counter ointments for shingles contain capsaicin, the substance that makes hot peppers hot. Like St. John's wort, capsaicin cannot be used on open lesions, so after they've cleared, use it to relieve the pain of postherpetic neuralgia, says Dr. Warnock. Capsaicin cream is available in a number of different strengths, ranging from 0.025 percent to 0.075 percent.

Capsaicin works by stimulating and then exhausting Substance P, the nerve-related transmitter in the skin that sends pain messages to your brain. After 2 to 3 days of applying capsaicin, you should begin to feel the pain subsiding. The cream itself is irritating to the skin, so start with a tiny amount. If a high-strength concentration burns too much, just switch to a lower strength, says Dr. Warnock.

Because capsaicin can burn the skin, however, he advises people to use it carefully. "I tell them to apply it four times a day to the affected area," he says. "You should always wear gloves when you apply it, and if you get it somewhere where you don't want it, don't try to wash it off with water. That just reactivates it and makes it worse. Instead, you can lessen the burning by rubbing the area with olive oil."

Add some licorice aid. Licorice also has strong antiviral properties. During the course of the infection, Dr. Warnock recommends taking 500 milligrams of standardized licorice extract in capsule form three times a day. If you take powdered licorice root in capsules, however, the dose should be 2,000 milligrams three times a day. Continue the treatment for 2 weeks after the lesions have healed, Dr. Warnock says.

Take licorice with caution, and don't take it at all if you are pregnant or nursing or if you have diabetes, high blood pressure, liver disorders, or kidney problems. In general, you shouldn't take high doses of licorice for more than 4 to 6 weeks unless you're under the supervision of a qualified health-care practitioner.

Battle back with C. High doses of vitamin C have been shown to keep the varicella zoster virus from replicating, according to some studies involving people who were given intravenous injections. There have not been any studies that showed similar effects with oral supplements. Dr. Warnock believes, however, that, with a daily dose of 10,000 milligrams of vitamin C, you can help keep the virus from taking hold. Dr. Warnock recommends five doses of 2,000 milligrams each, taken 3 hours apart. "The dosage goes beyond being a simple immune booster," he says. "The point is to interrupt the virus."

Dr. Warnock thinks vitamin C might prevent the virus from multiplying and spreading along the infected nerve. At the same time, vitamin C may ease inflammation in the nerve and lessen the outbreaks of the lesions, he says.

With a dose this high, you might experience an upset stomach and diarrhea, which are frequent side effects of excess vitamin C. If so, just reduce the dose until you reach a level that's more tolerable, says Dr. Warnock.

"Also, you need to take this treatment early in the infection," he says. "Once there are millions of virus particles floating around, it becomes a much harder task to keep them from reproducing."

Starve the virus. Varicella zoster belongs to a larger family of herpesviruses, all of which share an important characteristic: They multiply with the help of the amino acid arginine and are inhibited by another amino acid called lysine. Lysine may work by blocking the virus's ability to absorb and use arginine.

To keep shingles at bay, doctors advise, you should avoid arginine-rich foods, such as chocolate, legumes, and nuts, especially peanuts, and eat more foods that are rich in lysine, such as fish, tofu, eggs, lean beef, and lean pork.

You can also boost your lysine levels by taking a supplement. Dr. Warnock suggests taking 2,000 milligrams of lysine daily until the infection runs its course.

Shoulder Pain

Shoulder pain comes in lots of shapes and sizes. Some folks ache in their upper backs and some in the front of their shoulders, along the line from the top of the breastbone to the armpit. Still others hurt along the top, from their necks to the curve of their shoulders. The kind of pain varies, too, from a dull ache to a sharp, stabbing pain.

If you have shoulder trouble, even simple everyday activities like reaching up and putting the groceries in the cupboard can be tough. Moderating or stopping the offending activity—at least for a while—is the first step on the road to recovery. But in addition, here are some other ways to ease shoulder pain and help prevent a recurrence.

Exercise after your workout. "Shoulder pain often results from repetitive motion—whether it's caused by your job or by playing a sport such as tennis or softball," says Robert Stephens, Ph.D., chairman of the department of anatomy and director of sports medicine at the University of Health Sciences College of Osteopathic Medicine in Kansas City, Missouri.

"One of the best ways to remedy this problem, and help prevent it in the future, is to perform full range-of-motion stretching and strengthening exercises in order to compensate for these repetitive movements. For instance, if you have shoulder pain after playing tennis, perform some gentle stretching exercises such as rotating your arm inward and outward and doing slow, full arm circles (like the backstroke and crawl stroke) in both directions," says Dr. Stephens. "Stretching the muscles associated with the movement that's causing you the pain may help prevent muscle imbalances and ease the tension on the joints."

Use heat, but don't rely on it. Applying heat to a sore shoulder will help ease your pain, but it won't cure it.

"A heating pad is to shoulder pain what a microwave oven is to a bad sandwich: The sandwich tastes better warm, but if you let it cool down again, it'll taste just as bad as it did before you warmed it," says sports medicine specialist Charles Norelli, M.D., staff physiatrist at Good Shepherd Rehabilitation Hospital in Allentown, Pennsylvania. "In other words, you'll feel better while you have heat on your shoulder, but unless you fix the problem, you'll feel just as bad once you remove the heat."

When to See a Doctor

If pain, tightness, or limited range of motion in your shoulder interferes with everyday tasks, such as combing your hair or fastening bra hooks, and persists for more than 5 to 7 days, you should seek medical attention, advises Dan Hamner, M.D., a physiatrist and sports medicine specialist in New York City.

Wear a muffler. If you notice more shoulder pain in the winter, then Mother Nature might be more to blame than an active lifestyle.

"A lot of times, people get shoulder pain because they're breathing cold air. The pain they feel is really referred pain from the lungs' taking in freezing air," says A. J. Hahn, D.C., a chiropractor in Napoleon, Ohio, who specializes in natural remedies. "The answer is to wear a muffler or scarf during the cold months."

Stretch for Relief

All shoulder pain has two things in common—one bad and one good. On the negative side, it's extremely debilitating. Since you use your shoulders so frequently, if one of them hurts, you may wince as often as you smile. But on the positive side, you can fight shoulder pain with exercise by building up the joints.

"Human body joints, like cars, need maintenance," says Thomas Meade, M.D., orthopedic surgeon and medical director of the Allentown Sports Medicine and Human Performance Center in Pennsylvania. "There is no body version of motor oil, so we must think of these exercises as preventive maintenance for our bodies."

Try these simple stretches to alleviate any aches you have and to help prevent future pain.

Tug your towel. After you step out of your morning shower and dry off, turn your towel into an exercise tool for your achy shoulders, suggests Dr. Meade.

- Standing straight, hold one end of the towel with your right hand and let hang it down behind your back. Hold it so that your right fist is a few inches above your right shoulder.
- Reach behind your back with your left hand and grasp the other end of the towel.

- With your right hand, try to raise the towel as high as you can while resisting the upward pull by bearing down with your left hand.
- Hold for 10 seconds, then slowly lower your right hand and relax.
- Try this stretch four more times, then repeat on the other side.

Try to Find the Cause

All shoulder pain might hurt like the dickens, but not all the pain comes from the same source. To determine the probable cause of your problem, sports medicine specialist Charles Norelli, M.D., staff physiatrist at Good Shepherd Rehabilitation Hospital in Allentown, Pennsylvania, suggests you try these exercises.

- Hold your arm out and twist your wrist as though you were emptying a soda can, then raise your arm. If this causes pain, your problem is probably tendinitis.
- If the pain is in your right shoulder, grab your right elbow with your left hand and pull it across your body. If this causes pain, that might be a signal that something in the bone or muscle is getting in the way. This problem may be remedied with specific range-of-motion exercises and light weight lifting.

Dr. Norelli points out that any severe shoulder pain requires professional medical attention. Heart attack pain, for example, can sometimes be transferred to the shoulder. While these quick "diagnostics" can give you a clue in many cases, if the pain is severe, be sure to see your doctor for a more thorough examination.

Hug yourself. You can warm your shoulder muscles with this body hug, offered by Dr. Meade. He recommends doing this stretch twice a day to keep your shoulder muscles limber.

Stand straight and place your left forearm across your waist, with your left elbow bent at a 90-degree angle. Place your right forearm on top of your left so that your right hand cups your left elbow. Use your right hand to pull slowly and firmly on your left elbow for 20 to 30 seconds. Don't try to resist with your left arm. You should feel the muscles stretching in your shoulder and elbow joints. Switch arms and repeat.

Bring out the broom. There's no need for expensive gym equipment to keep your shoulders moving in all directions. Even a broom handle can help keep your shoulders supple.

Sit straight in a chair, your feet flat on the floor. With your arms straight, hold the broom handle in both hands, palms down, in front of your waist. Slowly lift your arms and raise the handle as high as you can—ideally, over your head. (If you have tendinitis, don't go higher than your shoulders.) Count to 5 or 10 and then lower the broom handle back to waist level. Try at least 15 repetitions twice a day.

"You should go to the point of feeling a little discomfort, but do not push it to the point of pain," advises Kim Fagan, M.D., a sports medicine physician at the Alabama Sports Medicine and Orthopedic Center in Birmingham.

Strengthen for Prevention

Shoulders need more strength training than most joints. "The shoulder's design is great for flexibility and range of motion, but it is lacking in stability," says Dr. Fagan. "For it to function properly, the surrounding muscles have to do their jobs well." She offers these stabilizing exercises to bolster the deltoid muscles, rotator cuff tendons, and shoulder blade stabilizers.

Soup up your shoulder. Grab a couple of cans of soup from the pantry and give yourself a workout before dinner.

Stand straight with your shoulders back. Your arms should be hanging at your sides with each hand holding a soup can.

Keeping your elbows straight and your palms facing the floor, slowly raise your arms to shoulder level. Hold for 5 seconds, then relax and slowly lower your arms. Repeat this lift four more times. Build up a little each day until you can hoist the cans 15 times per session.

Take cans in hand again. Before you put the soup away, try these moves, suggests Dr. Fagan. Hold one soup can with your arm hanging straight down at your side. Slowly and with controlled movements, swing the can back and forth like a pendulum. Be sure to keep your arm straight. For starters, try 25 swings with each arm three times a day. For variety, try making circular motions with the can. "The can holding is a little resistance training for the rotator cuff," explains Dr. Fagan.

Shrug and strengthen. Don't expect Arnold Schwarzenegger deltoids, but here is a series of easy exercises to ensure healthier shoulders, recommended by Michael Ciccotti, M.D., an orthopedic surgeon and director of sports medicine at the Rothman Institute at Thomas Jefferson University in Philadelphia.

Stand straight with your arms at your sides. Lift your shoulders for a count of two, then let them down on a count of two. Do 20 repetitions. Then try alternate left and right shoulder shrugs, repeating 20 times with each shoulder. Finish by moving both shoulders forward and then backward 20 times.

Sinus Pain

Our sinuses—eight little caves behind the eyes and nose—are defenders of our lungs. When everything's okay in there, the mucus that lines the sinuses acts like fly-paper, catching airborne enemies such as viruses, allergens, and dust before they can infiltrate our lungs. In addition to sifting out debris, these remarkable little recesses prepare air for our lungs in other ways, warming cool air, cooling hot air, and moisturizing air that's too dry.

Sinus problems arise when the sinus membranes swell, preventing the mucus from draining properly. Mucus buildup leads to blockage and pressure and results in sinusitis, which can be acute or chronic. Acute sinusitis has symptoms such as pain, nasal congestion, fever, and thick drainage from the nose over the course of 2 to 8 weeks. Chronic sinusitis, with many of the same symptoms—as well as sore throat, malaise, and poor sense of smell—can linger for months.

Since the sinuses are crowded tightly near your eyes and brain, it's important to control infection in that area before it spreads. See a doctor if you notice swelling around the eye, greenish mucus from your nose, or pain that lasts for more than 14 days after a cold starts. You may need antibiotics and other prescription drugs to clear up your sinuses, or even surgery if your problems are severe enough.

There are also a number of ways to ease sinus pain in your own home with simple remedies.

For Fast Relief

Flush them out. Doctors commonly recommend that you rinse out your nasal passages with salt water to clear out debris and infection when you have sinusitis and to help the area stay healthy the rest of the time.

Mix up a solution of ¼ teaspoon of salt and ¼ teaspoon of baking soda in 8 ounces of warm water, says Michael Kaliner, M.D., medical director of the Institute for Asthma and Allergy in Washington, D.C. With a bulb syringe, available at drugstores, squirt this solution up one nostril, then the other, until all 8 ounces have been used. Bend forward, your head over the sink. The solution may leak out your other nostril or down the back of your throat (if it does, just spit it out). You should do this twice a day, once in the morning and once at night, during a bout of sinusitis and once or twice a day as a preventive measure. Be sure to clean out the bulb with water after each use.

Alternatively, you can pump a saline spray, also available at drugstores, up into your nose, Dr. Kaliner adds.

Make it like a sauna in there. Another way to clean out your nasal passages is to breathe steam through your nose, Dr. Kaliner says.

There are several ways to get your sinuses steaming. An inexpensive method is to boil a pot of water, take it off the stove, and inhale the steam through your nose, he says. Make sure that you approach the rising steam cautiously, however, and don't let it scald you. Other ways to breathe in steam are to lean over a facial sauna device or simply take a hot, steamy shower.

Don't get dried out. To keep your sinuses draining well, don't allow yourself to get dehydrated. Make certain that you drink plenty of fluids—six to eight full glasses a day, says Lee Williams, M.D., associate professor of otolaryngology at Johns Hopkins University and author of *The Sinusitis Help Book*. This will help the mucous membranes lining your sinuses and nasal passages to stay moist, which in turn will make them more resistant to infection and sinus flare-ups.

Try a souper remedy. Mom may have been on to something when she ladled out bowls of hot chicken soup to treat your childhood colds, says Wellington Tichenor, M.D., a New York City internist and allergist specializing in the treatment of sinusitis. There is some evidence that it can help move mucus in your sinuses better than an ordinary hot fluid, though it's unclear how it works.

Towel off. Another way to improve sinus drainage, which may also reduce your pain, is to apply warm, moist heat to your face, Dr. Williams says.

For example, wring out a damp washcloth or folded towel in hot water from the spigot, then lay it over your nose, face, and cheeks. Make certain that the washcloth isn't hot enough to burn you. Reapply as soon as it begins to cool, and continue doing this for 5 to 10 minutes several times a day. Lying down with a dry towel over your face after the procedure keeps the area from cooling off too rapidly.

Don't take pain lying down. Sleeping elevated on a 7-inch-high sleeping wedge with a pillow on top of that will improve drainage and limit swelling in your sinuses, thereby reducing pain, Dr. Williams says. These wedges are available in some medical supply and department store catalogs, and most drugstores will order one for you.

It's better to lie on your "good side," with your affected sinus "up" in order to reduce swelling and improve its drainage, he says.

Work It Out

Even if you're tired and achy from sinusitis, a brisk walk or a light bike ride is wonderful for relieving sinus pain, says Alexander C. Chester, M.D., clinical professor of medicine at Georgetown University Medical Center in Washington, D.C. Although a little exercise is good, however, it doesn't necessarily follow that more is better. If you're really feeling lousy, don't exercise strenuously or for too long, says Dr. Chester. And don't try an exercise cure if you have a fever, he adds.

Pace it off. Relief may be as close as your front door. Whenever you feel especially stuffed up, put on your sneakers and head out for a leisurely stroll. Choose a fairly level course that will take you about 20 minutes to complete when you're going at a relaxed pace.

Scarf up for moisture. If it's chilly, use a scarf to cover your mouth and nose, Dr. Chester advises. This will help humidify the air and start the mucus running. Cram some tissues into your coat pocket—you'll need them.

Cycle your sinuses clear. Dig a bike out of the garage and take a spin around the neighborhood. Put it into a low gear, and pedal at a comfortable pace. "Your sinuses should open up shortly after beginning exercise," says Dr. Chester, so take some tissues along.

Ride inside. If you have a stationary bike and a humidifier, you can really unclog the works. Exercising in moist air will help loosen the mucus even more, says Dr. Chester.

Dodge the dry chill. During any season of the year, the best indoor environment for exercise is both humidified

and well-ventilated with outside air. "It's best to avoid exercising in air-conditioned health clubs because the air is
too dry and can make sinusitis worse," says Dr. Chester.

High-Altitude Pain Prevention

Inflate your sinuses. Some people may experience sinus
pain and ear discomfort at high altitudes, especially when
flying—and more so when descending—in a plane. This
happens especially if they have chronic sinus blockage or
chronic Eustachian tube blockage. In such instances, in-
flating your ears and sinuses repeatedly during flight will
prevent a partial vacuum in your ears or sinuses and possibly save you considerable discomfort.

To ward off this pain, Dr. Williams recommends that
you do the following exercise. Three times a minute
during takeoff and ascent, close your mouth, pinch your
nostrils shut and swallow, then immediately force air into
your sinuses and ears by blowing your nose with your nostrils still pinched shut. If you blow immediately after you
swallow, you don't have to blow hard to accomplish this.
A loud squeaking sound means that things were badly
blocked, making it even more important to keep doing it.

After the plane levels off, do this three times an hour
during the entire flight until you start descending. Then
again start puffing the air up into your ears, nose, and sinuses three times a minute once you start your descent to
land. Continue to do this until you land and for a while
afterward if your ears or sinuses still feel blocked. You
should not do this with a fresh cold, nor should you fly
with a cold either. If you do this procedure with a fresh
cold, you could force infection into your ears or deeper
into your sinuses.

Temporomandibular Disorder (TMD)

Wake up! Shower. Forget your briefcase as you rush out the door. Merge onto that parking lot called a freeway. Arrive late. Stain your shirt while guzzling coffee. Make some copies. Attend a meeting. Head home. Cook supper. Go to bed.

The stress producers in our daily lives are more prolific and intricate than the programming on cable TV. And stress is nasty stuff. Like excessive fat in our diets, it leads to a whole host of related problems ranging from heart disease and insomnia to colds and allergies.

Well, now you can add pain in the joints and muscles of your face—called temporomandibular disorder, or TMD—to the list of stress-related problems. When you have TMD, your jaw may lock when you try to open and close your mouth, and you may find it painful to chew. The pain and chewing difficulty may also be associated with a clicking sound. (See your dentist if you experience these symptoms or find that your ability to function normally is limited—if you cannot open your mouth wide enough to eat, for instance.)

It was dentists who named this painful condition TMD, after the temporomandibular joints, which are little jaw-operating hinges right in front of your earlobes. It might be that you've had a defect in the joint since you were born and some lifestyle factor has prompted the pain. Other things, too, can cause it, such as being socked in the jaw or suffering a head injury from a fall or an accident. And although stress often contributes to TMD, it can also be triggered if you spend long periods with your mouth open (during dental work, for instance), if you have poor posture, or if you grind your teeth.

"TMD can be tough to diagnose because so many of its symptoms are shared by other medical conditions," says Charles McNeill, D.D.S., professor in the department of restorative dentistry at the University of California, San Francisco, and director of the Center for Orofacial Pain in San Francisco. It's not unusual for TMD patients' complaints to include earaches and headaches as well as the more common jaw and facial pain.

Dentists often initially prescribe a self-care regimen that includes jaw exercises for TMD. In fact, if your dentist immediately suggests jaw surgery or wants to grind down your teeth, you should seek other opinions before you agree, says Dr. McNeill. "In all of the patients I have, only about 2 percent ever need surgery for TMD," he observes.

Among your alternatives—and certainly the first to try—is healing with motion. Exercise can relieve TMD pain in a number of ways. First, depending on the cause of your TMD, posture improvement might be a total cure. Or you might need to start doing jaw exercises that can help rebuild connective tissues and retrain uncoordinated jaw muscles. When you do these exercises regularly, they can rehabilitate tight, shortened muscles, enabling them to handle the daily rigors of chewing, yawning, and talking.

And, not least of all, exercise can help relieve stress. No matter what the root cause of your TMD or the events that worsen it, you'll help relieve that pain if you make some moves to relieve stress.

Workouts from the Neck Up

A number of neck exercises for TMD may be especially helpful. "I tell all of my patients to check for correct posture and tongue position and do one of the following neck exercises at least every 2 hours, and more often if they are really stressed or have a lot of jaw pain," says Bernadette Jaeger, D.D.S., associate professor of diagnostic sciences and orofacial pain at the University of California, Los An-

Make Eating a Pleasure Again

"Eating can be a challenge for people with TMD," says Patricia Rudd, director of physical therapy at the Center for Orofacial Pain in San Francisco. Here are her suggestions to restore your enjoyment.

Slow down. Eating more slowly helps prevent overtiring your jaw. It's the difference between running a mile and walking it.

Eat smaller meals. For a jaw with TMD, a full-course meal can be akin to a marathon. "Stop eating when your jaw starts to hurt," says Rudd. You can make your condition worse if you ignore the pain.

Go soft. Eating apples and other hard foods can intensify TMD pain. Switch to softer foods. Start off with vegetable soup instead of carrots and dip. Try grilled fish

geles, School of Dentistry. "Depending on how long you have been experiencing the pain, you should feel relief with these exercises if you do them consistently over a period of several weeks," she says.

Get it straight. If you jut out your chin and hunch your shoulders forward, as many of us do unconsciously, you're making the muscles around your mouth work harder because it's harder to keep your mouth closed. This extra effort puts extra strain on the temporomandibular (TM) joint. Although it may seem unrelated at first glance, correcting your posture is one of the most important ways to relieve jaw pain, says Dr. Jaeger.

For correct posture, your ears, shoulders, and hips should all be in a straight line, says Dr. Jaeger. You'll achieve that alignment if you move your shoulders back and allow them to relax. Then lift your chest, straighten

instead of grilled steak. Switch to peas and applesauce instead of broccoli and cauliflower. For dessert, go for frozen yogurt instead of gingersnaps.

"The idea is to give your jaw a rest," Rudd says. After you've followed the soft-food routine for a while, you might want to start eating foods that are slightly harder and build up from there. But always stop eating something if it becomes painful.

Keep it small. If you cut your food into small pieces, your jaw will have to do less work chewing. Cut finger foods into bite-size bits and place them near the back of your mouth so your molars do the work. Your front teeth should do as little biting off as possible, because that biting motion can irritate your TM joint, Rudd says.

your hips, and let your knees relax. In this position your neck and facial muscles, as well as your TM joint, do only the amount of work needed to hold your head up.

If you're not used to this posture, it may seem uncomfortable at first. And you might want to post some reminders around your home or work area; just a vertical line on a Post-it Note will do the trick. As you work at improving your posture, it will become second nature, says Dr. Jaeger. You may feel an immediate improvement in your jaw, or it might take several weeks.

Open your mouth and say "N." When you work at keeping your jaw closed—actually clenching or grinding your teeth—you'll need to try some tactics to unlock your jaw muscles. Putting your tongue in its proper place can help.

Just say the letter "N," says Dr. Jaeger. When you do, you put your tongue on the roof of your mouth behind your top front teeth. In the "N" position, your upper and lower jaws are slightly apart even if your lips are closed, she notes. When you start checking yourself, you might want to set an alarm or a signal on your computer (if you're near a workstation) that will remind you every 2 hours to check whether your tongue is in this position. Of course, when you eat or talk, your tongue is no longer in this position, but get used to returning to "N" when you finish.

Stretch it out. Here's a simple neck exercise recommended by Dr. Jaeger that will really help ease some of the tension that gets into your jaw. To position yourself for this exercise, find a chair with a hard seat, a straight back, and arms. Put your hands on the arms of the chair and hold that position while you straighten up, making sure that your ears are in line with your shoulders. Now you're ready to begin. Do the stretch once slowly.

- Inhale. As you exhale slowly through your nose, gradually lean your head to the left. Try to bring your ear as close to your left shoulder as you can without raising your right shoulder or rotating your head.
- When your ear is near your shoulder, hold the position for 30 seconds, breathing normally.
- Raise your head slowly and reverse direction, leaning your right ear toward your right shoulder.

Look around. Small muscles deep inside the neck can send you sharp reminders of TMD unless you stretch them out. By turning your head from side to side, you stretch some of those muscles and help relieve the tension stored there, says Dr. Jaeger. This exercise should also be done seated upright in a hard-bottom chair, but the chair doesn't have to have arms. Perform this routine once slowly.

- Sitting up straight with your upper body aligned, inhale. Slowly exhale through your mouth, simultaneously turning your head to the right and looking as far over your right shoulder as you can.
- Hold for 30 seconds, breathing normally.
- Face forward again, then pivot your head to look over your left shoulder.

Catch flies. Learning to open and close your mouth without stressing your TM joint can help reduce jaw pain, says Dr. Jaeger. This "fly-catching" exercise will also stretch the muscles that close your jaw and will help with jaw muscle coordination, she says. One tip: You may want to practice this maneuver in front of a mirror to make sure that you're opening your mouth in a straight line, not at an angle. Perform this routine one time through, slowly.

- Start in a good posture position, with your tongue in the "N" position to relax your jaw.

- Put your fingers on the TM joint, in front of each earlobe.
- Slowly open your mouth straight up and down, lowering your jaw as far as you can while keeping your tongue on the roof of your mouth. Hold this position for 30 seconds.

Rub it out. Massaging your chewing muscles can really help ease your pain, says Patricia Rudd, director of physical therapy at the Center for Orofacial Pain in San Francisco. Whenever your jaw hurts, put your fingers on your TM joints. Then gently rub those areas, using a circular motion. Continue for a few minutes, she says.

"I tell some of my patients to massage their chewing muscles in elevators, at traffic lights—wherever and whenever they feel pain from them," says Rudd. "It's a good technique because it relaxes the jaw muscles and improves local circulation." Just be careful not to rub so hard that you aggravate the joint pain, she cautions.

Spit it out. If you chew gum, you might irritate your TM joints and muscles tremendously, says Rudd. Gum chewing overtires the jaw muscles, she points out. The instant relief from jaw pain that you'll notice will make it worth giving up the gum.

Wrist Pain

People who work their wrists hard—guitarists, typists, and carpenters, for example—are at high risk for wrist pain. The wrist is a delicate network of tiny bones, nerves, tendons, and ligaments. Arthritis can attack there, and strains or sprains can make simple everyday tasks, such as opening a jar or even turning the pages of a book, quite painful.

The key to beating wrist pain is to make sure that your wrists are as limber and as strong as they can be. Experts suggest that you combine stretching exercises (to enhance your range of motion) and strengthening exercises (to build up the tendons, ligaments, and muscles in the wrist area).

"Remember to warm up your hands first. Hands must be warm in order to work correctly," says Robert Markison, M.D., a hand surgeon and associate clinical professor of surgery at the University of California, San Francisco.

Reach for a Warmup

There's nothing like a proper stretch to get the tendons, ligaments, and muscles in the wrist area warmed up, say doctors and physical therapists. Here are some handy stretches that may relieve and possibly prevent further wrist pain.

Revisit your childhood. Ask a five-year-old his age and he will likely declare "Five," raise his hand, and spread all five fingers as proof. The same gesture can be a curing stretch, says Thomas Meade, M.D., an orthopedic surgeon and medical director of the Allentown Sports Medicine and Human Performance Center in Pennsylvania. Here's how.

Place your hand out in front of you as if you were stopping traffic. With your arm extended, spread your fingers as far apart as possible. Hold that position for at least 20 seconds. Repeat it five times, then relax and do the same stretch with your other hand. "Your muscles and tendons won't remember this stretch unless you hold it for at least 20 seconds," says Dr. Meade. "You should be able to feel your muscles get more rubbery and stretchy with time."

Halt and stretch. You can use that crossing guard "Stop" pose for this stretch, too. First, extend one arm in front of you at shoulder level and parallel to the ground, your wrist bent and your palm facing out. Then use your other hand to gently pull back the fingers of your extended hand. Hold for 20 seconds, then relax. Repeat five times, then switch hands and repeat.

The goal is to feel the muscles, ligaments, and tendons stretching in your fingers, hand, wrist, and forearm, says Dan Hamner, M.D., a physiatrist and sports medicine specialist in New York City.

Grab for the door. All you need for this stretch is an imaginary front door, says Michael Ciccotti, M.D., an orthopedic surgeon and director of sports medicine at the Rothman Institute at Thomas Jefferson University in Philadelphia.

Extend your right arm in front of you with your palm facing the ground, then pretend that you are turning a

Try Wrist Resistance

A thick rubber band can actually be a piece of workout equipment. Try this rubber resistance regimen, suggested by Teri Bielefeld, P.T., a physical therapist and certified hand therapist at the Zablocki Veterans Affairs Medical Center in Milwaukee.

Extend your right arm in front of you, palm up. Slip a thick rubber band over the crease on the inside of your palm. Placing your left hand under your right hand, grab the other end of the rubber band. As your left hand slowly pulls the rubber band down, counter by trying to bend your right hand up at the wrist. Feel the resistance. Try 10 times and then repeat, switching hands.

Then turn your right hand palm down and do the same thing. As your left hand slowly tugs downward, try to flex your right hand up, once again using your wrist. Feel the resistance. Try 10 times, then switch hands and repeat.

"You're working on resistance with the wrist motion so that neither the wrist nor the rubber band wins," Bielefeld says.

doorknob slowly to the left, then slowly back to the right. Try 10 of these rotations, then switch hands and do 10 more. "This exercise helps make the joints in the wrist more supple," explains Dr. Ciccotti.

Think sink. Warm water can soothe aches in your wrists, says Jane Katz, Ed.D., professor of health and physical education at John Jay College of Criminal Justice at the City University of New York, world Masters champion swimmer, member of the 1964 U.S. Olympic performance synchronized swimming team, and author of *The New W.E.T. Workout*.

A Farewell to Wrist Pain

These exercises can help prevent further pain by building flexibility in your wrists, says Teri Bielefeld, P.T., a physical therapist and certified hand therapist at the Zablocki Veterans Affairs Medical Center in Milwaukee.

Wave goodbye to pain. This range-of-motion exercise is designed to stretch the muscles in the wrist area.

Extend your right arm straight in front of you with the palm down. Bend your wrist down, then raise it as if you were doing a slow-motion wave. Do 10 waves with each wrist three times a day, says Bielefeld.

Do the twist. For this flexibility builder, extend your right arm straight in front of you and cup your right elbow with your left hand. Keeping your right elbow still, rotate your right wrist, slowly turning your palm up and then down. Do this for 20 to 30 seconds and then repeat for a total of five repetitions. You should be able to feel the muscles in your arm twisting. Then switch arm positions and repeat with the other wrist. Try this exercise three times a day, suggests Bielefeld.

Submerge your hand wrist-deep in a sink full of warm water. Pivot your wrists to do 10 hand circles to the right, then 10 to the left.

This exercise improves the range of motion in your wrist and increases the flow of oxygen-carrying blood to your wrists and fingers, says Dr. Katz. "The beauty of exercising in water is that your muscles get resistance from all directions," she adds.

Play shadow games. Relive those childhood days of making shadow animals on your bedroom wall at night. This exercise mixes fun with flexibility, says Teri Bielefeld, P.T., a physical therapist and certified hand therapist at the Zablocki Veterans Affairs Medical Center in Milwaukee.

- Raise your right hand as if you were being sworn in to testify in court. Keep your fingers relaxed.
- Gently bend your right hand forward at the wrist so that your hand resembles a swan's head.
- Use your other hand to push down gently on the top of the "swan's head."
- Hold for 5 seconds, then gently bring your hand back into the starting position.
- Hold for 5 seconds. Repeat four times.

Arm Yourself with Strengthening Exercises

Once you have done stretches to limber up your wrists, step two is to try some exercises that make your wrists and forearms strong. Here are a few.

Tug on a towel. Roll up a hand towel, then grasp it with both hands. Keep your left hand still as you turn your right hand as though you were wringing out excess water, first in one direction, then the other. Repeat, turning with your left hand, says Mary Ann Towne, P.T., a physical therapist and director of rehabilitation and wellness services of the Cleveland Clinic Florida in Fort Lauderdale.

"When you wring a towel, you are both strengthening and stretching the muscles in your wrist," explains Towne.

Go fly fishing. Fly fishing is a good wrist-strengthening exercise as long as you don't overdo it, says Dr. Ciccotti. "It is a wonderful recreational sport as long as you prepare by doing some wrist stretches. The back-and-forth action flexes and extends the muscles. Using muscles rapidly requires strength and force. You are also stretching the joint capsule around your wrist."

Look, Ma, all hands. Try this imaginary hand-pedaling exercise. Extend both arms in front of you and pretend that your fingers are holding on to bicycle pedals. Making a forward circular motion with your arms, move the imaginary pedals forward. Make sure that you flex your wrists as you pedal. You should feel the muscles in your wrists, forearms, and elbows warming up, says Dr. Ciccotti. Gradually work up to 3 minutes of continuous exercise.

Index

Underscored page references indicate boxed text.